CASE STUDIES IN
IMMUNOLOGY

COMPANION TO IMMUNOLOGY FIFTH EDITION

JONATHAN BROSTOFF
MA DM(Oxon) DSc FRCP(Lond) FRCPath

Professor of Allergy and Environmental
Health
Centre for Allergy Research
Department of Immunology
University College London Medical School
London, UK

ALEXANDER GRAY
BSc MB BS

Department of Immunology
University College London Medical School
London, UK

DAVID MALE
MA PhD

Senior Lecturer in Neuroimmunology
Department of Neuroimmunology
Institute of Psychiatry
London, UK

IVAN ROITT
MA DSc (Oxon) Hon FRCP (Lond) FRCPath FRS

Emeritus Professor of Immunology
Director of Institute of Biomedical Science
University College London Medical School
London, UK

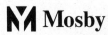 Mosby

London Philadelphia St Louis Sydney Tokyo

Senior Project Manager	**Linda Horrell**
Project Manager	**Elizabeth Payne**
Publisher	**Dianne Zack**
Managing Editor	**Louise Crowe**
Cover Design	**Greg Smith**
Illustration	**Danny Pyne**
Production	**Gudrun Hughes**
Index	**John Gibson**

Copyright © 1998 Mosby International Limited

Published by Mosby, an imprint of Mosby International Limited

Printed by JW Arrowsmith Limited

Text set in Galliard; captions set in Univers

ISBN 0 7234 2945 6

First published by Mosby, an imprint of Times Mirror International Publishers Limited, 1994, ISBN 0 7234 2052 1

Second edition published by Mosby, an imprint of Times Mirror International Publishers Limited, 1996, ISBN 0 7234 2214 1

For full details of all Mosby International Limited titles, please write to Mosby International Limited, Lynton House, 7–12 Tavistock Square, London WC1H 9LB, UK.

A CIP catalogue record for this book is available from the British Library.

Library of Congress Cataloging-in-Publication Data has been applied for.

Contents

Preface

In this new and enlarged edition, we have further increased the number and the scope of the case studies. The exciting discoveries in basic immunology, and cell and molecular biology, throw new light and understanding on the clinical manifestations of immunopathology in man and in animals. This knowledge must increase our chances of successful management and treatment of these diseases.

As always, our book of case studies is designed to put clinical 'flesh' on the 'skeleton' of basic immunology and to place immunological mechanisms within the framework of a clinical perspective.

We are absolutely of the opinion that immunlogy is relevant and indeed central to many diseases in both animals and man. Even if you, the reader, are not planning a clinical career, we hope that these case studies will provide you with a further perspective on the wide variety of immune-related diseases and perhaps add to your comprehension of the basic immunological mechanisms described in our fifth edition of *Immunology*.

Acknowledgements

We are grateful for the advice and comments on the case studies from the following colleagues and friends: Drs G Scott, S O'Connell, J Stanford, T Leslie, M Singer, J Garson, J Cambridge, R Mirakian, K Acland, J Gilkes, G Bothamley, V Novelli.

JB, AG

CASE 1

At 13 years of age, Steven was knocked off his bicycle by a car and was taken to his local hospital. On examination he had multiple minor lacerations to his left arm and leg but no evidence of fractures. Radiographs of his chest, pelvis and cervical spine were all normal. A brief mental state examination revealed a degree of confusion. This prompted an overnight stay in hospital for observation of suspected concussion.

During the night Steven became restless and complained of worsening abdominal pain. On examination he had a poor volume pulse and tachycardia. His jugular venous pulse was not visible and his blood pressure was 85/55 mmHg. Abdominal examination revealed bruising of the left upper quadrant and mild generalised tenderness with guarding. Blood was taken for immediate crossmatching and transfusion was performed. Despite giving him five units of whole blood his blood pressure did not rise substantially and he was taken to the operating theatre for laparotomy. At operation, blood was found in the peritoneal cavity and the source of the haemorrhage was identified as a ruptured spleen, which was removed. He required further transfusions post-operatively but recovered well.

The results of post-operative investigations are shown in *Figure 1.1*.

The thrombocytosis was an indication for early post-operative mobilisation. Steven was started on a prophylactic course of penicillin V, which he was advised to continue until the age of 20.

Ten years later Steven was seen by his GP with a productive cough and right sided chest pain. On examination he was obviously unwell with a tachycardia of 110 beats/min, a respiratory rate of 23/min and a temperature of 38.5°C. His blood pressure was 95/65 mmHg. He was admitted to hospital with signs of consolidation in the lower lobe of his right lung. A chest X-ray confirmed the diagnosis of lobar pneumonia, which resolved following intravenous cefuroxime. Blood cultures taken prior to treatment were found to have grown *Streptococcus pneumoniae*, a Gram-positive coccus. Bacterial vaccines were administered subcutaneously under prophylactic antibiotic cover following recovery.

QUESTIONS

1 What is the architecture of the spleen and how does this relate to its function?
2 How does the loss of this function predispose to infection?
3 What changes are seen in the cellular, immunoglobulin and complement profiles following splenectomy?
4 Are specific immunisations advisable following splenectomy?

Investigation	Result (normal range)
Haemoglobin (g/dl)	13.2 (after transfusion) (13.5–18.0)
White cell count (x 10⁹/l)	12.5 (4.0–11.0)
Neutrophil count (x 10⁹/l)	8.5 (2.0–7.5)
Platelet count (x 10⁹/l)	512 (150–400)
Blood film	Howell–Jolly bodies
	Target cells
	Siderocytes
	Normoblasts
Serum immunoglobulins	
IgG (g/l)	4.2 (5.4–16.1)
IgM (g/l)	0.1 (0.5–1.9)
IgA (g/l)	2.0 (0.8–2.8)
Serum	
Sodium (mmol/l)	141 (134–145)
Potassium (mmol/l)	4.2 (3.5–5.0)
Chloride (mmol/l)	102 (95–105)
Urea (mmol/l)	3.2 (2.5–6.7)
Creatinine (µmol/l)	120 (70–150)
Urine output	75 ml/hr

Fig. 1.1 Results of investigations.

■ **CASE 1** pp. 33–34, 237–240

ANSWERS

1 What is the architecture of the spleen and how does this relate to its function?

The spleen is a soft encapsulated organ 12 cm long and 7 cm wide in an average person. It lies beneath the ninth, tenth and eleventh ribs and is not usually palpable if it is of normal size. It has a rich blood supply from the splenic artery. The spleen has trabeculae but is not divided into discrete nodules. Two types of tissue are found on cross section (*Fig. 1.2*):

1) The red pulp consists of sinuses which contain macrophages that phagocytose older erythrocytes (normal life span around 120 days). It also acts as a pool of erythrocytes, platelets and granulocytes, which can be mobilised in times of need.

2) The white pulp is composed of lymphoid tissue that is largely arranged around central arterioles (branches of the splenic artery) as the periarteriolar lymphoid sheath (PALS). The PALS is organised in a concentric fashion:

i) The marginal zone consists of specialised macrophages, dendritic cells, natural killer cells and slowly circulating B cells. The terminal portion of the central arterioles, the penicillar arteries, are found in this zone and it is here that lymphocytes leave the circulation to enter the splenic tissue. They then migrate to either ii) or iii).

ii) The T cell area consists largely of interdigitating cells that express class II major histocompatibility complex antigen (MHC II) and present antigen to T cells. The central arterioles are also found here.

iii) The B cell area consists largely of follicular dendritic cells (which express the IgG receptor, FcγR and the complement receptor, CR1) presenting antigen to B cells. There are two degrees of organisation which reflect the degree of stimulation of the lymphoid tissue by antigen:

a) Primary unstimulated follicles – aggregates of unstimulated B cells.

b) Secondary stimulated follicles with a central germinal centre and surrounding mantle zone.

T and B cells are found in B and T cell areas respectively. This overlap presumably allows the contact dependent signals required for a humoral immune response to proceed.

In summary, the spleen has an important role as part of the phagocytic reticuloendothelial system and is a site for the presentation of antigen and subsequent clonal expansion of lymphocytes.

2 How does the loss of this function predispose to infection?

The spleen is particularly effective at removing encapsulated bacteria by phagocytosis. Bacteria, such as *S. pneumoniae*, become coated with IgG and the C3 component of complement. Macrophages express receptors for both these molecules, which enhances phagocytosis. Removal of the spleen compromises this function and therefore reduces the threshold level of infection required to cause significant clinical disease.

3 What changes are seen in the cellular, immunoglobulin and complement profiles following splenectomy?

The findings post-operatively in Steven's case (*Fig. 1.1*) are not unusual. The increase in neutrophils and platelets is common and usually transient. Mobilising the patient is necessary as prophylaxis against venous thrombosis. The red cell count is usually normal and Howell–Jolly bodies, target cells, sidero-cytes and normoblasts may be seen on the blood film. Serum IgG2 and IgM concentrations may be low as the splenic lymphocytes are major producers of these antibodies. Complement components may also be similarly reduced.

4 Are specific immunisations advisable following splenectomy?

Guidelines in the UK regarding immunisation or antibiotic prophylaxis are as follows. Some 50% of all infections in these patients are caused by *S. pneumoniae* and the administration of a vaccine consisting of capsular polysaccharides derived from pathogenic pneumococcal strains has been advocated for some time. It should be administered 2 weeks before splenectomy if possible, with reimmunization every 5–10 years. Antibiotic prophylaxis is continued after vaccination. This usually consists of penicillin twice daily. Recent recommendations also include *Haemophilus influenzae* type b (Hib) and meningococcal A and C vaccines.

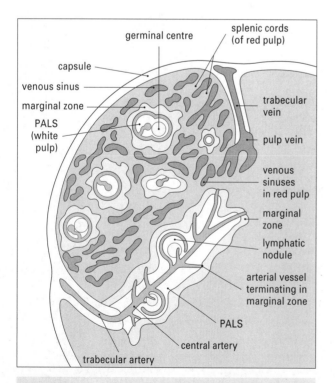

Fig. 1.2 Organisation of lymphoid tissue in the spleen.

■ CASE 2

Fifty-nine-year-old Mrs Quinn underwent elective sigmoid colectomy for recurrent diverticular disease. She had no other medical history of note and was fit and well before the operation. The procedure was carried out without incident and her immediate post-operative recovery was uneventful. Two days after surgery, however, she became acutely confused.

On examination she had a temperature of 38.5°C and a thready, radial pulse of 125 beats/min. Her blood pressure had dropped to 100/70 mmHg from an initial baseline of 140/90 mmHg and her jugular venous pulse was not visible. Her peripheral pulses were all present but her extremities felt cold. Examination of her abdomen was unremarkable with the wound uninfected and healing well.

On investigation her white cell count was $18.2 \times 10^9/l$, haemoglobin 11.8 g/dl and platelet count $130 \times 10^9/l$. Serum creatinine was mildly elevated. Samples of blood and urine were taken for culture, and she was started on cefuroxime, metronidazole and gentamicin for suspected septicaemia. Intravenous colloid was given to correct her hypovolaemia.

Over the next 12 hours her condition deteriorated. She became tachypnoeic and drifted into a semiconscious state. On examination she had widespread respiratory crackles and a radial pulse of 135 beats/min. Her blood pressure dropped to 90/50 mmHg. Arterial blood gas measurements showed a PaO_2 of 7.8 kPa *(normal range is >10.6 kPa)* and a $PaCO_2$ of 6.2 kPa *(normal range is 4.7–6.0 kPa)*, a pH of 7.157, a base excess of −8.9 and HCO_3^- of 17.3 on 60% oxygen by mask. She was immediately admitted to the intensive care unit.

On arrival she was intubated and intermittent positive pressure ventilation commenced. Further colloid was administered for hypovolaemia via a central venous line, and a pulmonary artery catheter was inserted. A chest X-ray was performed which showed bilateral interstitial lung infiltrates (*Fig. 2.1*).

A diagnosis of adult respiratory distress syndrome (ARDS) was made based on four criteria:
- A history of sepsis.
- A low $PaO_2/PaCO_2$ ratio.
- A non-raised pulmonary artery wedge pressure.
- Bilateral radiological lung infiltrates.

Intravenous colloids failed to improve Mrs Quinn's blood pressure, and as her cardiac output was elevated she was started on noradrenaline (a vasopressor agent). Intravenous low dose dopamine was given to improve renal and splanchnic perfusion, and a cause for her septicaemia was sought. A plain abdominal radiograph and an ultrasound scan did not reveal any abnormality. At laparotomy, purulent fluid was found in the peritoneal cavity and the colorectal anastomosis was found to have broken down. A defunctioning colostomy and peritoneal lavage were performed and Mrs Quinn was readmitted to intensive care. Three days post-operatively she developed a secondary chest infection and died shortly afterwards. Blood, urine and wound swab cultures were all negative but a culture of peritoneal fluid grew *Escherichia coli* (a Gram-negative bacillus of the coliform group) and *Streptococcus faecalis* (a Gram-positive coccus), both of which are normal bowel commensal bacteria.

QUESTIONS

1 What are endotoxins?
2 How do endotoxins mediate their effects?
3 What conditions are associated with ARDS?
4 What is the immunopathology of ARDS?

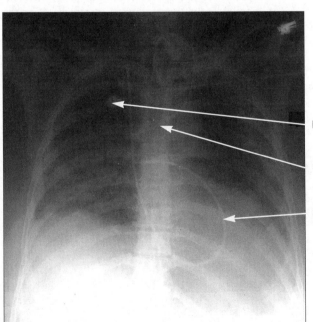

ECG lead

Venous catheter

Swann–Ganz catheter

Fig. 2.1 Chest X-ray showing bilateral interstitial lung infiltrates.

■ CASE 2   pp. 237–240

ANSWERS

1 What are endotoxins?

Endotoxins are structural components of bacterial Gram-negative cell walls, which are liberated only following cell death or lysis. They are complexes of phospholipids and polysaccharides, usually termed bacterial lipopolysaccharides (LPS). The lipid A component has been demonstrated to produce most of their toxic effects. Although their antigenicity varies between species, their biological effects are the same.

2 How do endotoxins mediate their effects?

Unlike exotoxins, endotoxins exhibit only weak antigenicity but they are still able to injure the parenchyma of various organs in severe sepsis. More significantly they are responsible for the activation of macrophages, which are important mediators of septic shock.

Macrophages release tumour necrosis factor (TNF) which acts on polymorphs and macrophages to mediate their activation, aggregation and adhesion to endothelial cells. TNF also stimulates the production of platelet activating factor (PAF), interleukin (IL)-1, IL-6 and the eicosanoids (thromboxanes, leukotrienes and prostaglandins) from neutrophils, macrophages, platelets and endothelial cells. These mediators have vasoactive properties and increase capillary permeability (*Fig. 2.2*).

Endotoxins also have a direct effect on neutrophils by increasing production and discharge of proteases and free oxygen radicals. They also directly activate the coagulation, fibrinolytic and contact dependent pathways. A consumptive coagulopathy results which can be manifested clinically as disseminated intravascular coagulation (DIC). This is characterised by an increased clotting time, a diminution of the platelet count and raised D-dimers. Both the classical and alternative complement cascades are also initiated.

The results of these processes are vasodilatation, hypotension and poor organ perfusion which may be beyond the reach of treatment.

3 What conditions are associated with ARDS?

The following conditions are common precursors of ARDS:
- Sepsis (bacteraemia, septicaemia).
- Trauma (head injuries, fat emboli).
- Localised infection (pneumonia).
- Aspiration (gastric contents, sea or fresh water).
- Haematological (haemorrhage, massive blood transfusion).
- Metabolic disorders (pancreatitis, uraemia).
- Others (inhaled toxins, drug overdose, radiation).

4 What is the immunopathology of ARDS?

It is believed that ARDS is triggered by an initial 'insult' related to one or more of the conditions listed above. Endotoxin liberation and/or complement activation result in macrophage activation and the release of TNF and IL-1. These have a variety of effects on different cellular and enzyme systems:
- Neutrophils: release of proteases, increased adherence and aggregation, and liberation of free oxygen radical scavengers.
- Platelets: aggregation, activation and release of eicosanoids.
- Endothelium: increased permeability and production of nitric oxide, increased arachidonic acid metabolism and release of prostaglandins, thromboxanes and leukotrienes.
- Activation of the coagulation pathway with concurrent fibrinolysis leading to generalised haemorrhage and the formation of microthrombi.

These factors combine to cause damage to the capillary endothelium and respiratory epithelium with sloughing of the cells lining the alveoli. The permeability of the endothelium and epithelium increases leading to interstitial and alveolar oedema with extravasation of red blood cells. The production of lecithin and sphingomyelin, the components of surfactant, is decreased following damage to the type II pneumocyte by proteolytic enzymes. The presence of fluid in the alveoli leads to a loss of function manifested as worsening hypoxaemia. A fall in lung compliance causes the lungs to become 'stiff'. Increasing ventilation pressures are therefore required to maintain adequate gaseous exchange. A fatal outcome in ARDS is not inevitable, but intensive therapy often fails to prevent a steady deterioration.

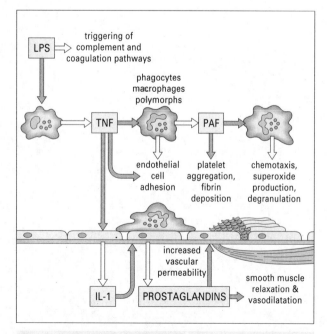

Fig. 2.2 Role of TNF in endotoxic shock.

■ CASE 3

Six-year-old John presented in the Accident & Emergency department with a 2-day history of malaise, fever, blood in his urine and a puffy face. He had no history of renal disease or abdominal trauma. Medical history of note was a sore throat some 12 days before, which had settled without a visit to his GP. His mother remembered that he had received the standard immunisation schedule (Appendix 4).

On examination John was febrile, had periorbital and ankle oedema, and his blood pressure was 130/90 mmHg. The skin on his face and trunk was peeling and he had a reddened tongue. The rest of his examination was unremarkable. Results of investigations are shown in *Figure 3.1*.

A diagnosis of post-streptococcal glomerulonephritis was made and John was started on benzylpenicillin. His fluid retention was controlled by restriction of salt and water intake and giving him loop diuretics. Within a week his blood pressure had dropped to 105/70 mmHg and there was no haematuria or proteinuria. Several weeks after presentation his C3 level had returned to normal. At follow-up he was well and had no signs of renal impairment.

QUESTIONS

1 What is the pathogenesis of post-streptococcal glomerulonephritis?
2 What is seen if a renal biopsy from this patient is stained with anti-IgG and anti-C3 antibodies conjugated to fluorescein?
3 What is the long-term prognosis of this condition?
4 Are all strains of Group A streptococci equally pathogenic?

Investigation	Result *(normal range)*
Haemoglobin *(g/dl)*	10.4 *(13.5–18.0)*
White cell count *(x 10^9/l)*	10.1 *(4.0–11.0)*
Platelet count *(x 10^9/l)*	285 *(150–400)*
Serum albumin *(g/l)*	31 *(35–50)*
C reactive protein *(mg/l)*	75 *(<5)*
Serum	
Sodium *(mmol/l)*	139 *(135–145)*
Potassium *(mmol/l)*	5.5 *(3.5–5.0)*
Chloride *(mmol/l)*	104 *(95–105)*
Urea *(mmol/l)*	8.5 *(2.5–6.7)*
Urine	
Visual inspection	Macroscopic haematuria
Glucose	Negative
Ketones	Negative
Microscopy	~5 white cells/ml
	Red cells
	Granular casts
Culture	<10^4 mixed organisms/ml
24 hr protein loss	2.1 g
Creatinine clearance	85 ml/min/1.73 m³
Culture from throat swab	Positive for *Streptococcus pyogenes*
Anti-streptococcal antibodies	
Streptolysin O (ASO)	Positive
DNAse B	Positive
Hyaluronidase	Positive
Serum C3 *(g/l)*	0.35 *(0.75–1.65)*
Serum C4 *(g/l)*	0.41 *(0.20–0.65)*

Fig. 3.1 Results of investigations.

■ CASE 3   pp. 237–239, 336–338

ANSWERS

1 What is the pathogenesis of post-streptococcal glomerulonephritis?

Post-streptococcal glomerulonephritis can occur at any age, but is most common in male children. The incidence of the disease, like that of rheumatic fever, has declined due to the widespread use of antibiotics in children with respiratory tract infections. The renal symptoms appear some 1–3 weeks after an acute infection, such as pharyngitis, with a group A β haemolytic streptococcus. Patients present with the nephritic syndrome characterised by oliguria, haematuria, proteinuria, diffuse oedema and hypertension. Renal biopsy shows acute diffuse proliferative glomerulonephritis. There is diffuse enlargement and increased cellularity of the glomeruli. The cellular changes are a mixture of increased numbers of endothelial and mesangial cells combined with infiltration of neutrophils and macrophages. Subepithelial electron-dense granular deposits are seen with electron microscopy.

2 What is seen if a renal biopsy from this patient is stained with anti-IgG and anti-C3 antibodies conjugated to fluorescein?

Immunofluorescence demonstrates that the electron-dense areas consist of deposits of IgG and C3, which implies that immune complexes have been deposited subepithelially. By implication it has been suggested that these complexes comprise streptococcal antigens bound with their specific antibodies. Experiments to identify bacterial antigens deposited in the glomeruli have produced conflicting results and it is not clear whether the complexes are formed in the circulation or *in situ*. Low circulating C3 and high anti-ASO antibody titres support an immune complex aetiology in this form of glomerulonephritis.

3 What is the long-term prognosis of this condition?

The prognosis is usually excellent if treatment is given rapidly. The glomeruli often return to normal within weeks, although the increased number of mesangial cells may persist for some months. The course may be more prolonged in adults, and a proportion sustain permanent renal damage. Most patients do not present with acute renal failure and treatment is usually supportive. Controlling hypertension is of importance in children to prevent the development of hypertensive encephalopathy which may occur with moderately elevated blood pressure levels.

It is worth noting that other infectious agents can cause glomerulonephritis, for example, *Staphylococcus aureus*, the Epstein–Barr virus and the malaria parasite. The most significant of these is glomerulonephritis in patients with infective endocarditis. This disease can be caused by a variety of organisms, including *Streptococcus viridans* and staphylococci.

4 Are all strains of Group A streptococci equally pathogenic?

Not all strains of Group A streptococci are equally pathogenic. Griffiths types 1, 4, 12, 25 and 49 have been noted to be nephritogenic with the other types not being associated with renal disease. No explanation has yet been found for this.

■ CASE 4

Sixty-one-year-old Mr Ranger had been a farmer and forester all of his working life and had always been fit. He went to his GP because of a bad headache, a stiff neck, and difficulty and pain when bending his head forward. He had also noticed difficulty in speaking, and eating had become more difficult because food and liquid dribbled from his mouth. His wife had to help him out of bed and out of his chair because of his stiff joints and his hands were particularly sore. He had recently suffered a bout of flu and thought that his current symptoms were related to this. His temperature was 38.6°C and he had some photophobia. Investigations at that time are shown in *Figure 4.1*.

The doctor suspected that he had developed an acute systemic disease involving the joints and decided to admit him to hospital.

On admission, there was evidence of arthralgia and a raised temperature, but only after further examination was bilateral facial palsy noticed as he had no facial asymmetry at rest. A lumbar puncture was immediately requested in view of the headache, photophobia and facial palsies.

A more detailed history was obtained. He regularly received tick bites while working as a forester. A month before admission he had noticed a faint erythematous rash on his leg around the site of a tick bite received 2 weeks earlier. The rash had expanded to 20 cm in diameter but had then cleared up without treatment.

A clinical diagnosis of Lyme disease was made and he was treated with benzylpenicillin. Approximately 6 hours after treatment had started his flu-like symptoms increased and he developed tachycardia and fever. These symptoms settled after 24 hours. Over the following 2 weeks his facial palsies and painful joints eased and he remained well 2 years later.

A strongly positive IgM and IgG antibody enzyme-linked immunosorbent assay (ELISA) to *Borrelia burgdorferi*, and an immunoblot pattern characteristic of an early disseminated infection, confirmed the clinical diagnosis of Lyme borreliosis after his discharge.

QUESTIONS

1 What are the stages of Lyme borreliosis?
2 Why did the patient feel worse shortly after starting the course of penicillin?
3 What is the explanation for the neurological problems? Could they be in part due to molecular mimicry?
4 Why might antibody tests for Lyme disease be non-specific?
5 Why do some of these patients develop chronic arthritis?

Investigation	Result (normal range)
Haemoglobin (g/dl)	14.8 (13.5–18.0)
White cell count (x 10⁹/l)	12.5 (4.0–11.0)
Lymphocyte count (x 10⁹/l)	7.9 (1.6–3.5)
ESR	42 mm/hr
Serum	
Sodium (mmol/l)	138 (134–145)
Potassium (mmol/l)	4.2 (3.5–5.0)
Chloride (mmol/l)	100 (95–105)
Urea (mmol/l)	6.2 (2.5–6.7)
Creatinine (μmol/l)	102 (70–150)
Blood glucose (mmol/l)	6.2 (<10.0)

Fig. 4.1 Results of investigations.

Investigation	Result (normal range)
CSF protein (mg/l)	0.75 (0.15–0.45)
CSF glucose (mmol/l)	3.0 (>60% of blood glucose)
CSF film	500 lymphocytes/mm³ No red blood cells seen No organisms present

Fig. 4.2 Results of investigations.

■ CASE 4   pp. 329, 229, 230

ANSWERS

1 What are the stages of Lyme borreliosis?

Lyme disease is caused by an infection with the spirochaete *B. burgdorferi*, which can be transmitted by the bite of an infected tick. Deer and other animals are the usual reservoir for the organism. Mr Ranger showed the classic progression of this disease.

- Stage 1 – early localised infection. This is called erythema migrans and the rash is seen originating from the site of the tick bite. Antigen from the organism may be found at the migrating margin of the rash.
- Stage 2 – early disseminated disease. Common clinical symptoms include multiple areas of erythema migrans, facial or cranial nerve palsies, small or large joint arthritis or carditis.
- Stage 3 – late persistent. Chronic large joint arthritis can occur in a small proportion of patients who had joint involvement during stage 2 of the disease. A skin condition (acrodermatitis chronica atrophica) and borrelia encephalomyelitis may occur.

2 Why did the patient feel worse shortly after starting the course of penicillin?

Penicillin, a bacterial agent, acts on the cell wall of the spirochaete releasing bacterial antigens both locally and systemically. Patients with Lyme disease have IgM and IgG antibodies in the circulation and in the cerebrospinal fluid (CSF). Antigen/antibody complexes are formed which fix complement and cause inflammation wherever the complexes 'precipitate out'. Patients may complain of joint pain and swelling, headache, rash (urticaria) and fever, which is characteristic. Bacterial products will also trigger cytokine release (including IL-1) from macrophages which elicits fever.

The immune complexes containing borrelia antigen are eventually cleared by the phagocytic system and the symptoms subside. This is a typical Type III hypersensitivity reaction.

3 What is the explanation for the neurological problems? Could they be in part due to molecular mimicry?

Patients with Lyme disease show symptoms indicative of both central and peripheral nervous system involvement. The infection can spread to the nervous system and present as nerve palsies. When the CSF is examined, there is often an increase in lymphocytes, a mildly elevated protein concentration and normal glucose levels. It may sometimes be possible to culture *Borrelia* from the CSF. However, the presence of DNA detected by polymerase chain reaction can confirm the infection more readily.

Chronic neurological problems probably result from direct infection of the central nervous system (CNS). Symptoms can improve after intravenous antibiotics, giving support to the claim that direct infection causes the symptoms.

Anti-neuronal antibody is present in a number of neurological diseases. Patients with Lyme disease with CNS involvement also have antibodies to axons, and experimental evidence shows that these antibodies can be absorbed out by *Borrelia* antigen and also by CNS tissue, suggesting a cross-reactivity between the organism and CNS tissue.

Anti-flagellin antibodies bind to axons but these are not necessarily specific for Lyme disease as they occur in other diseases where there has been infection by flagellated organisms. This does however provide a mechanism for molecular mimicry in this disease.

4 Why might antibody tests for Lyme disease be non-specific?

Most of the ELISA methods used for detecting Lyme disease use whole cell sonicates as antigen in the solid phase. The antibody response is against the flagellum and thus non-specific binding will occur in infections with other bacteria that contain flagella such as other *Borrelia*, *Treponema pallidum*, oral spirochaetes and other organisms. Cross-reactions can also occur in the presence of rheumatoid factor, anti-nuclear antibodies and in infectious mononucleosis. Western blotting gives a picture of the range of antigens to which the patient responds and can be used as evidence to confirm the specificity of the ELISA. It can be especially useful in serodiagnosis or exclusion of later Lyme disease because chronic infection gives a characteristic blotting pattern. There is a danger of Lyme disease being over-diagnosed if too great a reliance is placed on serology alone. The results should be interpreted in the light of symptoms and a detailed history of possible exposure. True positive results, consistent with a past infection, may also cause confusion when patients are being evaluated for another current illness. This is most likely to occur in patients from areas where *B. burgdorferi* is endemic.

5 Why do some of these patients develop chronic arthritis?

There is a higher rate of arthritic complications associated with Lyme disease acquired in North America than in Europe. This may in part be due to the strain of the organism that causes the infection. There are four distinct subspecies of *B. burgdorferi*, the main one strongly associated with arthritic complications. A very strong antibody response to its outer surface protein A (osp A) is found in patients with chronic Lyme arthritis. The European picture is more variable. *B. garinii* and *B. afzelii* are more common than *B. burgdorferi* and do not provoke strong osp A antibody responses. It is interesting that osp A is preferentially recognised by T-cell lines from patients with antibiotic treatment-resistant arthritis but is only rarely recognised by T cells from treatment-responsive arthritis.

Only a small proportion of infected patients, those who are HLA-DR4+, develop chronic antibiotic-resistant Lyme arthritis. The synovial lesions in chronic Lyme arthritis are similar to those seen in rheumatoid arthritis. Lyme arthritis must be one of the few forms of chronic arthritis where the exact cause is known.

■ CASE 5

Fifty-nine-year-old Mrs Jones was seen in Accident & Emergency after falling and injuring her right hip. On questioning she told of a 6-month history of backache, lethargy and weakness. She also reported fluctuating constipation, polyuria and polydipsia. She was postmenopausal but was taking hormone replacement therapy. Medical history consisted of three episodes of pneumococcal pneumonia in the past 2 years which had been treated successfully by her GP.

On examination, Mrs Jones had a swollen, tender and bruised right hip with 1 inch of true shortening of the right leg. She was clinically anaemic with pallor of her mucous membranes and nail beds and had a mild tachycardia. Her blood pressure was 135/85 mmHg. Her extremities felt cold but her peripheral pulses, including those of the right leg, were present. The rest of her examination was unremarkable. Results of investigations are shown in *Figure 5.1*.

X-ray of the hip showed the bone ends impacted and well aligned. Mrs Jones's fracture was initially managed conservatively with analgesia, fluids and bed-rest. Further investigations were performed, as a malignant lesion was suspected as the cause of the decreased bone density leading to the fracture (*Figs 5.2* and *5.3*).

A diagnosis of multiple myeloma was made and Mrs Jones was referred to an oncologist who prescribed a course of melphalan and prednisolone to control the malignancy. She responded to treatment and this allowed her fractured neck of femur to be repaired under general anaesthesia using a metal plate and nail.

Investigation	Result *(normal range)*
Serum immunoglobulins	
IgG *(g/l)*	59 *(5.4–16.1)*
IgM *(g/l)*	0.23 *(0.5–1.9)*
IgA *(g/l)*	0.45 *(0.8–2.8)*
Electrophoresis of serum proteins	A monoclonal peak in the γ region identified as IgG of the kappa type
Immunoelectrophoresis of a monoclonal protein band found in urine and blood	Kappa Bence–Jones protein
Serum β_2 microglobulin *(mg/l)*	4.2 *(1.2–2.4)*
Bone marrow biopsy	Plasmacytosis >28%

Fig. 5.2 Results of further investigations.

QUESTIONS

1 What is Bence–Jones protein?
2 What is the pathology of multiple myeloma and how is the diagnosis made?
3 Why has Mrs Jones had recurrent pneumonia?
4 Why is Mrs Jones anaemic?

Investigation	Result *(normal range)*
Haemoglobin *(g/dl)*	10.4 *(11.5–16.0)*
MCV *(fl)*	74.6
Blood film	Normocytic, normochromic red cells
White cell count *(x 10⁹/l)*	7.3 *(4.0–11.0)*
Platelet count *(x 10⁹/l)*	135 *(150–400)*
ESR	88 mm/hr
C reactive protein	40 *(<5)*
Serum albumin *(g/l)*	28 *(35–50)*
Serum	
Sodium *(mmol/l)*	141 *(134–145)*
Potassium *(mmol/l)*	4.3 *(3.5–5.0)*
Calcium (total) *(mmol/l)*	2.98 *(2.12–2.65)*
Chloride *(mmol/l)*	96 *(95–105)*
Urea *(mmol/l)*	15.6 *(2.5–6.7)*
Creatinine *(µmol/l)*	195 *(70–150)*
X-ray of pelvis and upper femurs	Complete transverse extracapsular fracture of the neck of the right femur through an area of decreased bone density

Fig. 5.1 Results of investigations.

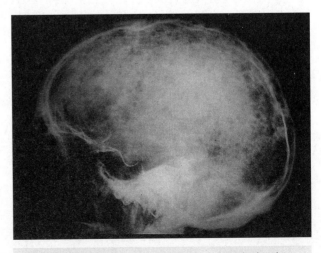

Fig. 5.3 Lateral skull X-ray showing multiple 'punched out' osteolytic lesions.

■ **CASE 5**   pp. 71–78, Chapter 20

ANSWERS

1 What is Bence–Jones protein?

Plasma cells synthesise a larger amount of immunoglobulin light chains than heavy chains. Whole immunoglobulins are not excreted by the kidney because their molecular weight is too high (IgG 146 kDa, IgM 970 kDa), but light chains (22 kDa) are found in the urine. Under normal circumstances, light chains are polyclonal in specificity, reflecting their synthesis by many different plasma cells. Bence–Jones proteins are free monoclonal light chains and therefore reflect their origin from a single antigen-specific plasma cell clone. A particular plasma cell is capable of synthesising only either kappa or lambda light chains. This explains the presence of only kappa chains in Mrs Jones's blood and urine.

2 What is the pathology of multiple myeloma and how is the diagnosis made?

Multiple myeloma is a neoplastic proliferation of plasma cells or their precursors within the bone marrow. The malignant proliferation of the cells is responsible for the bone lesions and the excess production of immunoglobulin, which is usually IgG or IgA (*Fig. 5.4*). This excess immunoglobulin is referred to as paraprotein. The aetiology and pathogenesis of multiple myeloma is unknown but excess IL-6 production has been implicated.

Diagnosis is based on a triad of findings:
- Bence–Jones protein in the blood and/or urine.
- Multiple osteolytic lesions of the bones.
- The presence of increased numbers of abnormal plasma cells or their precursors in the bone marrow. A plasmacytosis of >20% is used in making the diagnosis, but if all the cells are demonstrably of one light chain class, then a lower percentage

(around 12%) is acceptable. Paraproteins alone are not of value diagnostically as they are found in other conditions. Elevated serum β_2-microglobulin levels are associated with a poor prognosis. The mean survival from diagnosis is around 2 years.

Multiple lytic lesions and osteoporosis in multiple myeloma predispose to pathological fractures, most frequently of the wedge compression type found in the spinal column. Light chains are metabolised by cells of the proximal renal tubules but the excess found in multiple myeloma causes renal tubular necrosis and cast formation. A degree of renal failure is therefore common.

3 Why has Mrs Jones had recurrent pneumonia?

Patients with multiple myeloma have an increased susceptibility to bacterial infections, particularly pneumococcal pneumonia in the early stages of the disease, and sepsis and Gram-negative urinary tract infections in the later stages. This state is caused by a decrease in the production of normal immunoglobulins of all classes and is believed to originate from suppression of normal plasma cells by the malignancy.

4 Why is Mrs Jones anaemic?

Anaemia is found in the majority of patients with multiple myeloma at some point in the course of the disease. Anaemia is frequently normocytic and normochromic and is typically refractory to iron, folate and vitamin B12 treatment. The cause of the anaemia is loss of bone marrow because of tumour infiltration and the suppression of normal marrow by tumour cell secretions. The excess production of light chains is also associated with red cell haemolysis.

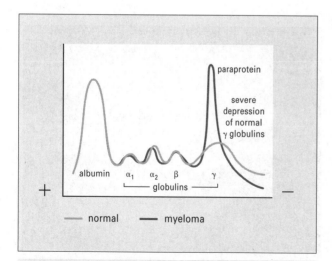

Fig. 5.4 Densitometry traces of serum protein electrophoresis from a normal subject and a subject with multiple myeloma.

Serum protein	Urine light chain type	% of patients
IgG	—	30
IgG	+BJκ	10
IgG	+BJλ	10
Total IgG		50
None	BJκ only	12
None	BJλ only	12
Total light chain		24
IgA	+BJκ	4
IgA	+BJλ	4
Total IgA		20
IgD	+BJκ	1

Fig. 5.5 Types of whole immunoglobulins and light chains in a series of multiple myeloma patients.

■ CASE 6

Rashmi, a 5-year-old girl, was seen in a haematology clinic with a 6-week history of worsening malaise, lethargy and anorexia. Her GP had seen her some 3 weeks previously and had diagnosed pharyngitis, which was treated with oral amoxycillin. Despite this, the infection had not cleared and Rashmi still had a persistent cough. Over the past week she had developed aching pains in her back and limbs which had failed to respond to oral analgesics. Within the past few days a purpuric rash had appeared on her left thigh. There was no history of haemoptysis or chest pain and there were no episodes of bleeding, or any gastro-intestinal or urinary symptoms.

Rashmi was born at 41 weeks and was the third child in the family. She had no history of recurrent or persistent infections or ill health. Her mother remembered her receiving the standard immunisation schedule and an additional BCG vaccination because of a family history of tuberculosis. She had no developmental difficulties and was shortly due to start school. Her brother and sister and both parents were fit and well.

On examination, Rashmi was between the 25th and 50th centiles for height, but between the 3rd and 10th centiles for weight. Her temperature was 37.2°C and her radial pulse was 98 beats/min. She appeared pale and was clinically anaemic. She was not jaundiced but her cervical, axillary and inguinal lymph nodes were palpable. A respiratory examination did not demonstrate any crackles or wheezes, and a cardiovascular examination was normal. Abdominal palpation revealed hepatosplenomegaly, but no tenderness or other masses. Rashmi's pharynx was also clearly inflamed and her tonsils were enlarged. Bleeding was observed from several sites along the gums. A neurological examination did not reveal any cranial or peripheral nerve lesions and optic fundoscopy was normal. Her chest X-ray was also normal. The results of investigations are shown in *Figure 6.1*.

A diagnosis of common, L1, acute lymphoblastic leukaemia (ALL) was made. Initial treatment was aimed at restoring red cell, platelet and neutrophil counts with transfusions. Remission was achieved using three agents: once weekly vincristine for 4 weeks, L-asparaginase twice to four times weekly for 4 weeks, and oral prednisolone daily for the same period. Consolidation therapy was carried out using 6-mercaptopurine, methotrexate, vincristine and prednisolone. Cranial prophylaxis was also administered in the form of cranial radiation and intrathecal methotrexate. Maintenance therapy of oral 6-mercaptopurine and methotrexate continued over a 2-year period.

Treatment was successful and at a follow-up 3 years after diagnosis, Rashmi was well and needed no further therapy.

QUESTIONS

1 What is acute leukaemia and how does it present?
2 How can the immunophenotyping of malignant cells aid in the diagnosis of ALL?
3 What prognostic indicators are of value in ALL?

Investigation	Result *(normal range)*
Haemoglobin *(g/dl)*	7.8 *(11.5–16.0)*
White cell count *(x 10⁹/l)*	12.3 *(6.8–10.0)*
Neutrophils *(x 10⁹/l)*	0.5 *(2.0–7.5)*
Eosinophils *(x 10⁹/l)*	0.32 *(0.4–0.44)*
Monocytes *(x 10⁹/l)*	0.1 *(0.2–0.8)*
Total lymphocytes *(x 10⁹/l)*	5.9 *(2.0–4.1)*
T lymphocytes *(x 10⁹/l)*	4.5 *(2.7–5.3)*
B lymphocytes *(x 10⁹/l)*	2.0 *(0.6–1.4)*
Blast cells	Elevated
Platelets *(x 10⁹/l)*	25 *(150–400)*
Serum immunoglobulins	All normal
Antibody response to infection CMV, VSV, measles	Negative
Serum	
Sodium *(mmol/l)*	133 *(134–145)*
Potassium *(mmol/l)*	3.3 *(3.5–5.0)*
Chloride *(mmol/l)*	102 *(95–105)*
Creatinine *(μmol/l)*	75 *(70–105)*
Calcium (total) *(mmol/l)*	2.41 *(2.12–2.65)*
Phosphate *(mmol/l)*	1.65 *(0.8–1.45)*
Culture	
Throat	β haemolytic streptococcus
Nose	*Staphylococcus aureus*
CSF from lumbar puncture	3 lymphocytes/mm³ No blast cells
Bone marrow aspirate blast cell analysis	
Cell size	Small
Cytoplasm	Scanty
Nuclear shape	Regular
Nuclear chromatin	Homogeneous
Nucleoli	Small
Immunological phenotyping of blast cells	
Nuclear Tdt	Positive
HLA-DR	Positive
CD10	Positive
CD19	Positive
sCD22	Positive
cIg	Positive
sIg	Negative
CD2	Negative
cCD3	Negative
CD7	Negative
Genetic analysis of blast cells	No aberrations

Tdt = terminal deoxynucleotidyltransferase; prefix c = cytoplasmic; prefix s = surface.

Fig. 6.1 Results of investigations.

■ **CASE 6**   pp. 273–283

ANSWERS

1   What is acute leukaemia and how does it present?
The acute leukaemias are a group of haematological malignancies characterised by the clonal expansion of immature haemopoietic cells (blast cells) which accumulate in the bone marrow and blood. They can be broadly classified into acute lymphoblastic leukaemia (ALL), thought to arise from early cells in the lymphoid series, and acute myeloid leukaemia (AML) where the cell of origin is likely to be of the myeloid or pluripotent stem cell lineage.

The incidence of ALL reaches a peak of 7/100 000 at 3–4 years of age but thereafter falls rapidly to around 0.5/100 000. ALL is the commonest malignancy in children. In contrast, the incidence of AML rises steadily with age to 15/100 000 at 70 years. Presentation is linked to marrow dysfunction caused by the excessive expansion of the monoclonal blast cells. Anaemia is a common finding manifested as malaise, lethargy and dyspnoea. Patients, who are usually neutropenic, are susceptible to infections which are often caused by normal commensal flora. Viral infections (e.g. herpes simplex) are also frequent. Platelet numbers are decreased and patients may present with spontaneous bruising and haemorrhages. Symptoms can also arise from leukaemic infiltration of organs, for example, deposits in bone cause dull pain and tenderness. Lymphadenopathy, hepatosplenomegaly and gingival infiltration are also common findings. Spread to the CSF may occur, particularly in ALL.

2   How can the immunophenotyping of malignant cells aid in the diagnosis of ALL?
Blast cells in ALL are initially classified morphologically using a variety of criteria including cell size and cytoplasmic and nuclear features. The L1 type, which makes up the majority of childhood ALL, consists mainly of small cells with scanty cytoplasm and a regular nucleus. L2, which is usually found in adults, is characterised by large cells with moderate quantities of cytoplasm and irregular nuclei. The L3 type, with large cells, moderate cytoplasmic content and regular nuclei, is associated with mature B-cell disease.

Immunophenotyping is carried out using monoclonal antibodies to cellular components. The antigenic profile can be used to determine the lineage of the blast cells (*Fig. 6.2*). Typing leukaemic cells is not an esoteric exercise; it allows residual cells to be identified following treatment and also aids in determining the prognosis. Changes in chromosome number and structure in blast cells, found in over 80% of patients with ALL, are also assessed routinely. Examples of aberrations include a translocation from chromosome 9 to 22, known as the Philadelphia chromosome. This abnormality is found in only 3% of childhood ALL, but occurs in 90% of chronic myeloid leukaemia cases. Translocations are often associated with particular subtypes of ALL. The t1; 19 (q23; p13.3) translocation, for example, is often found in pre-B-ALL.

3   What prognostic indicators are of value in ALL?
The most important factor in influencing the prognosis in ALL is the achievement of an initial remission and its duration. The prognosis is significantly worse in children below the age of 1 year and is worse in males, regardless of age. This is in part because testicular relapse occurs in 10% of males, whilst ovarian relapse is rare. So called 'bulky disease', characterised by lymphadenopathy, massive splenomegaly or a significant mediastinal mass, is also associated with a poor outcome.

The total white cell count prior to treatment is the single most valuable prognostic indicator. Other laboratory indices are also of value. Both the L2 and L3 morphologies have a poorer outcome, with the L3 group faring the worst. Null, T- and B-cell variants, as determined by immunophenotyping, carry a poorer prognosis than the common and pre-B-cell types. Certain genetic aberrations also influence prognosis. The t1; 19(q23; p13.3) translocation, for example, has a poor outcome.

Phenotype	Cell marker									
	Nucleus Tdt	HLA-DR	CD10	CD19	sCD22	cIg	sIg	CD2	cCD3	CD7
Null ALL	+	+	−	+ > −	−	−	−	−	−	−
Common ALL	+	+	+	+	−	−	−	−	−	−
Pre-B-ALL	+	+	+	+	+	+	−	−	−	−
B-ALL	−	+	− > +	+	+	na	+	−	−	−
T-ALL	+	−	−	−	−	−	−	+	+	+

Tdt = terminal deoxynucleotidyltranferase; Ig = immunoglobulin; prefix s = surface; prefix c = cytoplasmic; na = not applicable.

Fig. 6.2 Phenotypic markers in acute lymphoblastic leukaemia.

■ CASE 7

John was born at term after an uneventful pregnancy and was well for the first 18 months of life. He received the standard immunisation schedule for his age and had no growth or developmental problems. From the age of 2 years he suffered from frequent upper respiratory tract infections, several of which required oral amoxycillin. He was twice admitted to his local hospital with a diagnosis of bronchiolitis and on one occasion a right middle lobe pneumonia was diagnosed. He was also referred to the ENT team because of recurrent otitis media associated with ongoing tonsillitis.

At 3 years of age, John was seen by his GP with unilateral purulent rhinorrhoea associated with facial pain, a post-nasal drip, fever and malaise. On examination he was obviously unwell with a tachycardia of 125 beats/min and a temperature of 38.8°C. His left nostril was encrusted with exudate which could also be clearly seen over his red and swollen nasal turbinates. He was admitted to hospital where a frontal skull X-ray demonstrated a fluid level in the left maxillary sinus, confirming a diagnosis of acute maxillary sinusitis. Intravenous ampicillin resolved the infection over a period of 4 days.

At 5 years of age, he developed a perennial nocturnal cough with wheezing and breathlessness. A peak flow measurement was below the normal range for his age and height. A diagnosis of allergic asthma was made and he was started on inhaled sodium cromoglycate (a mast cell membrane stabilising agent) and salbutamol (a β_2-adrenoceptor agonist). Typical hay fever symptoms of watery rhinorrhoea and itchy conjunctivitis started the following summer and were treated with oral anti-histamines.

The following winter he was admitted twice into hospital with acute severe asthma complicated by bacterial chest infections. The results of investigations following one of these episodes are shown in *Figure 7.1*.

A diagnosis of selective IgA deficiency was made and John was prescribed continuing therapy for his asthma and respiratory tract infections. Recurrent tonsillitis was an indication for the removal of his tonsils some months later.

Investigation	Result (normal range)
Haemoglobin (g/dl)	15.2 (13.5–18.0)
White cell count (x 10⁹/l)	15.8 (6.8–10.0)
Neutrophils (x 10⁹/l)	13.8 (2.0–7.5)
Eosinophils (x 10⁹/l)	0.67 (0.4–0.44)
Total lymphocytes (x 10⁹/l)	4.3 (2.7–5.4)
T lymphocytes (x 10⁹/l)	2.4 (2.7–5.3)
B lymphocytes (x 10⁹/l)	1.0 (0.6–1.4)
Serum immunoglobulins	
IgG (g/l)	18.9 (4.9–16.1)
IgG1 (g/l)	14.3 (5.6–11.3)
IgG2 (g/l)	3.6 (0.4–4.0)
IgG3 (g/l)	0.6 (0.3–0.8)
IgG4 (g/l)	0.62 (0.14–0.95)
IgM (g/l)	2.4 (0.5–2.0)
IgE (IU/ml)	235 (3–150)
IgA (g/l)	0.025 (0.4–2.0)
Antibodies made to immunisations	All present
Skin prick tests	Grade (0–5)
D. pteronyssinus*	3+
Cat	3+
Mixed grass	3+
Egg	3+
Milk	2+
Sweat sodium†	57 mmol/l

* House dust mite
† Sweat sodium concentration >70 mmol/l is diagnostic for cystic fibrosis in a child

Fig. 7.1 Results of investigations.

QUESTIONS

1 What is the aetiology and pathogenesis of selective IgA deficiency?
2 What clinical associations exist with this condition?
3 What other immunoglobulin abnormalities may be found with a low IgA and how do they alter the clinical presentation?
4 What precautions should be taken when giving a blood transfusion to a patient with IgA deficiency?

■ CASE 7   p. 286

ANSWERS

1 What is the aetiology and pathogenesis of selective IgA deficiency?

Selective IgA deficiency is the most common cause of primary immunodeficiency in the UK with an incidence of 1 in 700, although it is rare in Japan at 1 in 18 500. The majority of cases arise sporadically but familial forms have been described which are responsible for up to 20% of cases in some populations. Familial analyses have identified two putative modes of inheritance; autosomal dominant and autosomal recessive. Several HLA associations with IgA deficiency have also been reported. The HLA-B8, -DR3 haplotype, which also has a strong association with coeliac disease, is more common in patients with IgA deficiency.

Two types of IgA exist in man, IgA1 and IgA2. IgA1 is the predominant subclass in serum and is found mainly as a monomer. IgA2 is the predominant immunoglobulin in secretions (e.g. saliva, gut and respiratory mucous) and occurs as a dimer with the two Fc regions of the antibodies bound together by a J chain. Secretion across the mucosa is mediated by a specific secretory component which binds to a cell receptor. The overwhelming majority of patients who are IgA deficient fail to produce both subclasses but isolated deficiencies have been reported.

It could be postulated that the genes coding for IgA are abnormal in deficient patients but chromosomal analyses have failed to demonstrate deletions within the genes coding for the IgA heavy chains or the region responsible for switching production of immunoglobulin to IgA. Furthermore, deficient patients have a normal number of B cells expressing membrane-bound IgA. It has been suggested that, despite cell surface expression, these cells are unable to differentiate into IgA secreting plasma cells. Genetic similarities have been observed with common variable immunodeficiency. Both conditions may be caused by autosomally transmitted gene defects with limited penetrance.

2 What clinical associations exist with this condition?

Three types of disorders are associated with selective IgA deficiency:

- Recurrent bacterial and viral infections of the respiratory and gastrointestinal tract, attributed to the lack of secretory IgA. The majority of patients have an increased level of serum and secretory IgG and IgM, and this may explain why most IgA deficient patients are asymptomatic. Those without this compensatory mechanism are more prone to infections.
- The incidence of allergic disease is higher in symptomatic IgA deficient patients than the normal population at around 25%. A possible explanation is that decreased mucosal clearance of allergen allows greater exposure but this has not been demonstrated. Such patients are often more resistant to therapy for their allergies.
- IgA deficiency is associated, to varying degrees, with autoimmune disease (*Fig. 7.2*). There is also an increased incidence of patients who are asymptomatic but who have autoantibodies such as rheumatoid factor (see Case 31) and anti-DNA and anti-nuclear antibodies (see Case 28). Many patients also have anti-IgA antibodies which are usually of the IgG class but may be IgD, IgE or IgM. There is also an increased incidence in these patients of certain inflammatory conditions (*Fig. 7.2*).

3 What other immunoglobulin abnormalities may be found with a low IgA and how do they alter the clinical presentation?

A proportion of patients with selective IgA deficiency also have IgG2 and/or IgG4 subclass deficiencies. Inherited immunoglobulin heavy chain gene defects have been demonstrated in certain families. Although in a normal subject these immunoglobulins comprise only 12% and 5% respectively of the total serum IgG, they have a particular role to play in the immune response. IgG2 deficiency in particular is associated with an inability to respond to capsular polysaccharide antigens such as those found on *Streptococcus pneumoniae* and *Haemophilus influenzae*. Both organisms can cause respiratory tract infections and meningitis. It is still unclear whether the combination of IgA and IgG subclass deficiencies is associated with a greater risk of infection than IgA deficiency alone but anecdotal evidence suggests this is the case.

4 What precautions should be taken when giving a blood transfusion to a patient with IgA deficiency?

Patients with IgA deficiency may have anti-IgA antibodies. If so, they are at risk of severe, and sometimes fatal, anaphylactic reactions from the administration of whole blood.

If a patient needs blood to correct anaemia, packed and washed red cells are recommended. Ideally the patient should be transfused with his or her own, stored blood or ABO/Rh matched units from another IgA deficient patient. The efficacy of intravenous gammaglobulin therapy in treating IgA deficiency is questionable and has inherent risks.

Systemic autoimmune diseases
  Systemic lupus erythematosus
  Rheumatoid arthritis
  Dermatomyositis

Organ-specific autoimmune diseases
  Insulin dependent diabetes mellitus
  Myasthenia gravis
  Autoimmune thyroiditis
  Pernicious anaemia
  Autoimmune haemolytic anaemia

Intestinal diseases
  Crohn's disease
  Ulcerative colitis
  Coeliac disease

Fig. 7.2 Autoimmune and inflammatory diseases associated with selective IgA deficiency.

■ CASE 8

Peter was born at term after an uneventful pregnancy and weighed 4.1 kg at birth. Whilst in the neonatal unit, he developed a vesicular rash on his torso and face. Bacterial and viral culture of swabs from mother and child were negative but Peter was given parenteral antibiotics and acyclovir for a suspected herpes simplex infection. He was discharged 10 days later but was readmitted at 8 weeks of age with a widespread vesicular, weeping and encrusted skin rash, fever and poor feeding.

On examination, he was febrile and had a purulent discharge from his left external auditory meatus, diagnosed as otitis externa. Cultures of the discharge grew *Staphylococcus aureus* and *Escherichia coli*. Swabs taken from affected areas of the skin also grew *S. aureus*. Parenteral cefotaxime was used to control the infections and scrupulous aural toilet was also instituted. Whilst in hospital he developed oral candidiasis which was treated with nystatin. He was eventually discharged on antibiotics and antifungal agents.

At 10 months of age, Peter was seen in Accident & Emergency with a tender mass in his left axilla which was diagnosed as axillary adenitis. The flocculent mass required surgical drainage and parenteral flucloxacillin. The causal organism was again identified as *S. aureus*. At this visit his weight and height were on the 3rd centile and a degree of developmental delay was noted. He had not yet started to speak and was unable to stand. Results of investigations from this admission are shown in *Figure 8.1*.

A diagnosis of hyperimmunoglobulinaemia E-recurrent infection syndrome was made based on a history of recurrent *S. aureus* infections, extremely elevated serum IgE and positive anti-*S. aureus* IgE antibodies. Over the next 2 years Peter was seen in hospital with recurrent cold staphylococcal abscesses, otitis media and adenitis and was prescribed daily prophylactic flucloxacillin. At 2 years of age, he developed a right lower lobe pneumonia; the causal organism was again identified as *S. aureus*. Despite the use of parenteral flucloxacillin, a right sided pneumatocoele developed that was later complicated by a pneumothorax. At this visit, delay in fine motor, general motor and language skills was noted. The results of skin prick tests to common allergens performed during this episode, and serial IgE measurements for the first 2 years of life, are shown in *Figure 8.2*.

QUESTIONS

1 What features characterise hyperimmunoglobulinaemia E-recurrent infection syndrome?
2 What is the pathogenesis of this disorder?
3 What conditions are associated with excessive or deficient production of IgE?

Investigation	Result (normal range)
Haemoglobin (g/dl)	9.7 (13.5–18.0)
White cell count (x 10⁹/l)	20.1 (6.4–11.0)
Neutrophils (x 10⁹/l)	18.0 (2.0–7.5)
Eosinophils (x 10⁹/l)	0.31 (0.4–0.44)
Total lymphocytes (x 10⁹/l)	0.9 (2.7–5.4)
Serum immunoglobulins	
IgG (g/l)	12.2 (3.0–15.8)
IgM (g/l)	1.6 (0.4–2.2)
IgE (IU/ml)	51 800 (<100)
IgA (g/l)	0.98 (0.15–1.3)
Lymphocyte response to *in vitro* stimulation with phytohaemagglutinin	Normal
Nitroblue tetrazolium test	Normal dye reduction
In vitro incubation of leucocytes with *S. aureus*	Normal bacterial killing compared with controls
Anti-*S. aureus* IgE	Positive

Fig. 8.1 Results of investigations.

Investigation	Result
Skin prick tests	Grade (0–5)
D. farinae	3+
Cat	3+
Dog	0
Cockroach	2+
Mixed grasses	0
Wheat	3+
Egg	3+
Milk	3+
Serum IgE	
8 weeks	150 mg/l
10 months	245 mg/l
12 months	29 mg/l
16 months	65 mg/l
20 months	59 mg/l
24 months	61 mg/l

Fig. 8.2 Results of serial indices for the first 2 years of life.

■ **CASE 8** p. 286

ANSWERS

1 What features characterise hyperimmunoglobulinaemia E-recurrent infection syndrome?

The hyperimmunoglobulinaemia E-recurrent infection syndrome is a primary immunodeficiency syndrome characterised by recurrent staphylococcal abscesses and highly elevated serum IgE. A similar condition, first described in 1966, was named 'Job's syndrome' after the biblical character whom Satan 'smote....with sore boils, from the sole of his foot unto his crown'. Both males and females may be affected, with 50% having a family history of hyper-IgE. This suggests an autosomal dominant mode of inheritance with variable penetrance.

Patients usually present in infancy with recurrent infections caused by *Staphylococcus aureus* and, less frequently, *Candida albicans*, *Haemophilus influenzae* and *Streptococcus pneumoniae*. Skin infections, typically abscesses but occasionally cellulitis, are found in all patients. The abscesses are often 'cold', that is they are not associated with an inflammatory response. Staphylococcal pneumonia leads to the formation of pneumatocoeles. Other common infections include sinusitis and otitis media.

Chronic dermatitis, found in the majority of the patients, does not have a typical atopic distribution. Skin prick tests, which can be carried out from infancy onwards, are often positive for common food and inhalant allergens such as wheat, egg, house-dust mite and cat. Coarse faces, characterised by a broad nasal bridge and prominent nose, are seen in approximately 70% of cases, although this finding is not present at birth. Osteopenia with apparently normal calcium and phosphate metabolism leading to pathological fractures is also common.

Serum IgE is extremely high with normal IgG, IgM and IgA. IgD levels are often elevated. Total white cell numbers may be normal or elevated with eosinophilia a consistent finding.

2 What is the pathogenesis of this disorder?

Despite much speculation, the primary defect in hyperimmunoglobulinaemia E-recurrent infection syndrome is unknown. It has been hypothesised that the elevated IgE found in these patients may be caused by excess IL-4 - production but this remains unproven. The relationship between hyper-IgE and immunodeficiency is also unclear.

Some authors have reported a defect in neutrophil chemotaxis in these patients but this is not found in all subjects. Depressed delayed cutaneous hypersensitivity to *C. albicans* is a feature in 50% of subjects. However, the majority have decreased *in vivo* lymphocyte responses to *C. albicans* and tetanus toxoid despite normal responses to phytohaemagglutinin (PHA). Staphylococcal-specific IgE, once believed to be pathognomonic for the syndrome, has also been found in a proportion of patients with atopic dermatitis.

3 What conditions are associated with excessive or deficient production of IgE?

See *Figure 8.3*.

Increased IgE

Atopic disease
  Asthma
  Allergic rhinitis
  Atopic dermatitis
  Food allergy

Parasitic disease
  Hookworm
  Schistosomiasis
  Ascariasis

Infectious disease
  Allergic bronchopulmonary aspergillosis
  HIV-1 infection
  Infectious mononucleosis
  Pertussis

Immunodeficiency disease
  Hyperimmunoglobulin E syndrome
  Wiskott–Aldrich syndrome
  DiGeorge syndrome
  Selective IgA deficiency
  Nezelof's syndrome

Skin disease
  Pemphigoid

Other conditions
  IgE myeloma
  Rheumatoid arthritis
  Cystic fibrosis
  Nephrotic syndrome
  Cigarette smoking
  Bone marrow

Decreased IgE

Severe combined immunodeficiency (SCID)
X-linked agammaglobulinaemia
Transient hypogammaglobulinaemia of infancy
Hyper-IgM
Ataxia telangiectasia
Familial IgE deficiency
Primary biliary cirrhosis

Fig. 8.3 Conditions associated with excessive or deficient production of IgE.

■ CASE 9

Alex was born at term after an uneventful pregnancy. Delivery was normal and at birth he weighed 4 kg. He did not require any resuscitation and had no anatomical abnormalities. His first few months of life were without incident but at 6 months he developed an upper respiratory tract infection that became complicated by *Haemophilus influenzae* sinusitis. He was treated in hospital with cefotaxime and recovered well. Within a month he was seen again by his doctor with a 2-day history of worsening fever and inadequate feeding. On examination he was irritable and dehydrated with a temperature of 38.5°C. His left tympanic membrane was inflamed but not perforated. A diagnosis of acute otitis media was made and he was admitted to hospital for parenteral antibiotic therapy and rehydration. A throat swab revealed the causal organism to be *H. influenzae*.

Within 48 hours of being admitted, Alex's condition deteriorated. He became increasingly drowsy and developed apnoeic episodes. A broad infection screen was immediately undertaken to find the cause. The results of these investigations are shown in *Figure 9.1*.

A diagnosis of acute bacterial meningitis was made based on the immediate findings in the cerebrospinal fluid (CSF), and a course of parenteral cefotaxime was started. His condition stabilised after 24 hours and he was discharged 5 days later. The otitis media did not clear fully and a further course of antibiotics was required to clear the infection.

At 12 months Alex was found to have a red, tender and swollen arm. A diagnosis of cellulitis was made and he was successfully treated with benzylpenicillin. At 15 months he was admitted to hospital with severe diarrhoea and failure to thrive. Stool culture revealed the causal organism to be *Giardia lamblia* and prolonged antibiotic therapy was again necessary to clear the infection. At this visit his height and weight were noted to be below the 3rd centile and his teeth were abnormally decayed for his age.

Alex's mother confirmed that he had received the standard immunisation schedule. No abnormal reactions had occurred after any immunisation. His older sisters aged 3 and 5 years had normal growth patterns and no history of recurrent or refractory infections. The results of investigations are shown in *Figure 9.2*.

A diagnosis of X-linked agammaglobulinaemia (Bruton's disease) was made and Alex was started on intravenous IgG replacement therapy. The immunoglobulin was obtained from a large pool of donor serum using ethanol fractionation, and administered at 3–4 week intervals. Members of his family were advised to attend for genetic counselling, which was aided by the use of a gene probe test for the deficiency. At a follow-up appointment several years later Alex was well and only one chest infection was reported since diagnosis.

QUESTIONS

1 What clinical features are found in X-linked agammaglobulinaemia (XLA)?
2 What is the molecular and genetic basis of XLA?
3 Why was Alex well for the first few months of life?

Investigation	Result *(normal range)*
Haemoglobin *(g/dl)*	14.7 *(13.5–18.0)*
White cell count *(x 10⁹/l)*	15.2 *(6.4–11.0)*
Blood glucose *(mmol/l)*	8.1 *(<10.0)*
Serum	
Sodium *(mmol/l)*	147 *(134–145)*
Potassium *(mmol/l)*	4.7 *(3.5–5.0)*
Chloride *(mmol/l)*	102 *(95–105)*
Creatinine *(μmol/l)*	120 *(70–150)*
Chest X-ray	Normal
Urine microscopy	~5 white cells/ml
Culture organisms	<10⁴ mixed/ml
Blood culture	Negative
CSF from lumbar puncture	
Appearance	Turbid
White cells *(polymorphs/mm³)*	2500
Protein *(mg/l)*	0.62 *(0.15–0.45)*
Glucose *(mmol/l)*	4.5 *(>60% of blood glucose)*
Gram stain	Gram-negative bacilli
Culture	Positive for *H. influenzae*

Fig. 9.1 Results of investigations.

Investigation	Result *(normal range)*
Haemoglobin *(g/dl)*	14.4 *(13.5–18.0)*
White cell count *(x 10⁹/l)*	8.2 *(6.8–10.0)*
Neutrophils *(x 10⁹/l)*	6.2 *(2.0–7.5)*
Eosinophils *(x 10⁹/l)*	0.31 *(0.4–0.44)*
Total lymphocytes *(x 10⁹/l)*	3.2 *(2.7–5.4)*
T lymphocytes *(x 10⁹/l)*	3.15 *(2.7–5.3)*
B lymphocytes *(x 10⁹/l)*	Very low, almost undetectable
Serum immunoglobulins	
IgG *(g/l)*	0.31 *(3.0–15.8)*
IgM *(g/l)*	0.03 *(0.4–2.2)*
IgE *(IU/ml)*	Not detected *(<100)*
IgA *(g/l)*	Not detected *(0.15–1.3)*
Antibodies made in response to immunisations	Not detected

Fig. 9.2 Results of investigations.

■ CASE 9   pp. 286–287, 168

ANSWERS

1   What clinical features are found in X-linked agammaglobulinaemia (XLA)?

XLA is characterised by extremely low circulating numbers of B lymphocytes with decreased or absent serum immunoglobulins. IgG levels are usually below 2 g/l with the other classes very low or undetectable. Occasionally the IgE levels are normal. Pre-B cells are found in normal numbers in the bone marrow of XLA patients suggesting a block in differentiation as the cause of the defect. Milder variants of the disease with greater numbers of B cells are rare.

Affected individuals usually present in the first year of life with recurrent infections caused by *Streptococcus pneumoniae*, *Haemophilus influenzae* and β haemolytic streptococci. Pneumonia, bronchitis, pharyngitis, sinusitis and otitis media are all common and often do not respond promptly or adequately to antibiotic therapy. Bacterial meningitis and septic arthritis are also common; the latter may be caused by unusual organisms such as *Ureaplasma urealyticum* (a causal organism of urethritis in adults). Chronic diarrhoea from *Giardia lamblia* infection is a frequent cause of failure to thrive in these infants.

In general, viral infections are handled normally by XLA patients, with three notable exceptions:

- Live attenuated polio vaccine or wild virus may cause paralysis and therefore vaccination should be avoided.
- Enteroviruses (e.g. echovirus 11) may cause chronic meningoencephalitis.
- Hepatitis viruses may cause severe chronic active hepatitis (see Case 32).

Rapid treatment of infections is vital as an adjunct to regular gammaglobulin infusions. The latter may also be added to the treatment of acute infections.

2   What is the molecular and genetic basis of XLA?

The genetic locus of XLA has recently been mapped to the Xq22 region on the long arm of the X chromosome. The area was sequenced and found to be highly homologous to members of the src-related tyrosine kinase family. Tyrosine kinases, which phosphorylate tyrosine residues, exist in two forms: those which span the cytoplasmic membrane and therefore have a receptor function, and those which are cytoplasmic. Bruton's tyrosine kinase, btk, is a member of the latter class.

It is now clear that aberrations within the btk gene, which has 19 exons, produce XLA, and several point mutations and deletions have been described in different families. To date the exact function of btk has not been elucidated but its relationship with other protein kinases found in association with the B-cell antigen receptor suggests that it may play a role in receptor signalling.

The structure of the B-cell antigen receptor and its putative relationship to cytoplasmic structures can be seen in *Figure 9.3*. The receptor complex is composed of two substructures. The first, which binds antigen, is a membrane bound immunoglobulin, usually of the IgM or IgD class. These differ from their secretory counterparts in having a transmembrane region at the C terminus to facilitate cell binding. The second, which has signal transduction capability, consists of a disulphide linked heterodimer with either α and β or α and γ subunits.

Blk, lyn, fyn, lck (which are all src-protein kinases) and Syk (Ptk72^{syk}) are associated with the B-cell antigen receptor and become activated when antigen is bound. These kinases phosphorylate a variety of intracellular proteins which have putative roles in cellular activation. As yet, the precise interactions between the receptor and effector pathways remain unclear.

It has recently been demonstrated that btk interacts with fyn, lyn and blk. It is possible therefore that btk plays a role in the antigen receptor signalling pathway that results in B-cell activation. Aberrations within btk could conceivably affect this process and block immunoglobulin synthesis. Recent evidence suggests that a delay or block in the development of pro-B cells to pre-B cells occurs in XLA.

3   Why was Alex well for the first few months of life?

Maternal IgG crosses the placenta from 16 weeks of gestation onwards and provides a protective level of immunoglobulin in the infant for 6–9 months (see Appendix 2a and 2b). Complications are therefore expected only after maternal antibody has disappeared, at which stage the child has little or no humoral protection. Many infants have a 'dip' in serum immunoglobulins at 6 months as the maternal antibody level drops and endogenous production rises. Transient hypogammaglobulinaemia of infancy occurs when the infant fails to produce IgG at this age. It can usually be distinguished from XLA by the presence of IgM, IgA, IgE and IgD, although occasionally there is also a temporary deficiency of IgM and IgA. Most of these patients do not require treatment with gammaglobulin.

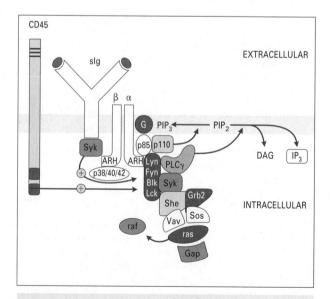

Fig. 9.3 Structure of the B-cell antigen receptor.

CASE 10

David was born at 37 weeks after an uneventful pregnancy. At birth he was cyanosed and required oxygen from the first few minutes of life. He was born with abnormal external features including micrognathia, large slanted eyes and low set prominent ears with notched pinnae. Within the first 36 hours of life he developed muscle tetany and convulsions. The results of investigations at this time are shown in *Figure 10.1*. The tetanic episodes were treated with intravenous calcium gluconate and were followed up with a low phosphorus diet, calcium supplements and high doses of vitamin D.

Over the next few days David developed tachypnoea and deep central cyanosis. On examination he had a harsh systolic murmur at the left sternal edge. The results of further investigations are shown in *Figure 10.2*.

A diagnosis of DiGeorge syndrome was made based on the following findings:
* Cardiac anomalies – tetralogy of Fallot* in this case
* Dysmorphic facial features
* Absence of thymic shadow on X-ray
* Hypocalcaemia

The following features confirmed the diagnosis:
* Very low T lymphocyte numbers
* Poor lymphocyte response to PHA
* The presence of a deletion on chromosome 22.

David's condition did not improve and by 2 months he had developed persistent oral candidiasis and diarrhoea. He was underweight for his age and his cardiovascular status remained unaltered. Cardiac surgery was delayed and a decision was taken to perform a foetal thymus transplant as soon as a donor became available. The thymus was obtained from a 12-week-old foetus, which was removed as an ectopic tubal pregnancy. The tissue was dissected and transplanted peritoneally within 2 hours. A white cell count taken some weeks later showed an increase in cell numbers but at 3 months he developed *Pneumocystis carinii* pneumonia, which proved fatal. An autopsy examination confirmed an absent thymus, a lack of T lymphocytes in the paracortical areas of lymph nodes and the cardiac anomalies.

*Tetralogy of Fallot consists of the following cardiac abnormalities:
* A ventricular septal defect
* Pulmonary stenosis
* An over-riding aorta
* Right ventricular hypertrophy (not present in David)

QUESTIONS

1 What is DiGeorge syndrome and how is it inherited?
2 What role does the thymus play in immune development?
3 To what infections was David especially prone?
4 Why did David have hypocalcaemia?

Investigation	Result (normal range)
Haemoglobin (g/dl)	14.2 (>16.0)
White cell count (x 10⁹/l)	5.2 (6.4–11.0)
Serum	
Sodium (mmol/l)	139 (134–145)
Potassium (mmol/l)	3.9 (3.5–5.0)
Chloride (mmol/l)	99 (95–105)
Creatinine (µmol/l)	82 (70–150)
Calcium (total) (mmol/l)	1.56 (2.12–2.65)
Phosphate (mmol/l)	1.26 (0.8–1.45)
Blood glucose (mmol/l)	6.8 (<10.0)
Parathyroid hormone (µg/l)	0.05 (0.1–0.73)
Chest X-ray	Absent thymic shadow

Fig. 10.1 Results of investigations.

Investigation	Result (normal range)
Haemoglobin (g/dl)	14.8 (13.5–18.0)
White cell count (x 10⁹/l)	6.7 (6.4–11.0)
Neutrophils (x 10⁹/l)	4.2 (2.0–7.5)
Eosinophils (x 10⁹/l)	0.26 (0.4–0.44)
Total lymphocytes (x 10⁹/l)	0.5 (2.7–5.4)
T lymphocytes (x 10⁹/l)	0.3 (2.7–5.3)
B lymphocytes (x 10⁹/l)	0.3 (0.6–1.4)
Lymphocyte response to *in vitro* stimulation with phytohaemagglutinin	Very low
Serum immunoglobulins	
IgG (g/l)	12.6 (2.4–8.8)
IgM (g/l)	0.15 (0.02–2.10)
IgE (IU/ml)	0.7 (0.3–20)
IgA (g/l)	0.01 (0.1–0.5)
Arterial blood gases	
PaO₂ (kPa)	7.8 (>10.6)
PaCO₂ (kPa)	5.8 (4.7–6.0)
Oxygen saturation	82%
Electrocardiogram	Normal
Echocardiogram	Ventricular septal defect (VSD) and an over-riding aorta
Doppler ultrasound scan	Pulmonary stenosis and blood flow through the VSD of the heart
Chromosomal analysis by fluorescent *in situ* hybridisation of gene probes	Sub-microscopic deletion in the proximal area of the long arm of chromosome 22

Fig. 10.2 Results of further investigations.

■ CASE 10   p. 290

ANSWERS

1   What is DiGeorge syndrome and how is it inherited?

DiGeorge syndrome (DGS) is a developmental disorder of the third and fourth pharyngeal pouches caused by deficient migration of neural crest cells. Patients have abnormalities of the face and ears, parathyroid insufficiency, congenital heart disease and thymic hypoplasia or aplasia. It is the thymic insufficiency that is responsible for the increased susceptibility to infection found in these individuals.

Up to 95% of patients with DGS have deletions within chromosome 22 at the 22q11 region. A small number of cases arise from deletions on chromosome 10. Recent work has shown that other related conditions are caused by similar defects in this area. It has been suggested that DGS is not a distinct disease but is part of a wider clinical spectrum of 22q11 associated disorders. The acronym CATCH 22 has been proposed to encompass the spectrum of Cardiac defects, Abnormal facies, thymic hypoplasia, Cleft palate and Hypocalcaemia seen in patients with such aberrations.

A few familial clusters of DGS have been identified but the majority of cases appear to arise sporadically. The familial clusters are also associated with chromosome 22q11 deletions. With the availability of genetic analysis the question of counselling parents with DGS offspring arises. Although the risk of passing on the 22q11 deletion is 1 in 2, many patients with the aberration do not develop significant cardiac or immunological dysfunction. The low risk should therefore not hinder parents considering further offspring.

2   What role does the thymus play in immune development?

The thymus is a critical tissue in the development of the immune system. Haemopoietic stem cells from the foetal liver and bone marrow migrate to the embryonic thymic rudiment and seed the thymus throughout life. The thymus provides a site for division and differentiation of these stem cells into T lymphocytes and is also largely responsible for selection of the T-cell repertoire by positive and negative mechanisms.

Developing T lymphocytes within the thymus undergo T cell receptor (TCR) gene rearrangements and express TCR at a low level. At this stage the cells also express both the CD4 and CD8 markers and are therefore termed double positive. Those double positive cells which recognise antigen presented by self major histocompatibility (MHC) molecules are positively selected, and mature into single positive CD4 or CD8 T lymphocytes which express TCR at a high level. Those which do not meet this criterion are deleted by programmed cell death (apoptosis). This process is termed positive selection.

T cells which recognise self antigens bound by MHC molecules also undergo apoptosis. The timing of this event in the developmental pathway of T cells is variable and depends on the type of cell presenting the antigen, the avidity of cell-cell binding and the availability of antigen. This process is termed negative selection.

The vast majority of cells (95%) are deleted by these processes. Those that are selected leave the thymus and are available for antigen driven clonal expansion.

3   To what infections was David especially prone?

Patients with DGS have an increased susceptibility to a variety of infectious agents. Typically, they can present with recurrent pneumonia (including *Pneumocystis carinii* pneumonia) and chronic sinusitis caused by *H. influenzae*. Oral candida and persistent diarrhoea are common. Viral infections are frequently caused by herpes simplex and zoster viruses.

4   Why did David have hypocalcaemia?

The parathyroid glands are also derived from the third and fourth pharyngeal pouches, the third providing the inferior glands and the fourth, the superior. The DiGeorge abnormality is therefore usually complicated by primary hypoparathyroidism manifested as hypocalcaemia, hyperphosphataemia and low or absent parathyroid hormone.

■ CASE 11

Six-month-old Oscar was seen in Accident & Emergency after two episodes of bloody diarrhoea. He had not vomited any blood but his mother felt that Oscar had been irritable and off his food. He had also developed a rash on his forehead and cheeks over the past couple of days. He had become increasingly drowsy over the past 5 hours and his mother was clearly anxious.

Oscar was born at 39 weeks after an uneventful pregnancy. He weighed 3.2 kg at birth and had an unremarkable neonatal period. Aged 12 weeks, he developed a worsening productive cough and a diagnosis of right lower lobe pneumonia was made. Between the ages of 12 and 18 weeks he was seen three times in Accident & Emergency with otitis media, which was treated with intravenous ampicillin. This had not resolved and as a result he had a perforated right tympanic membrane that was discharging purulent fluid. At 22 weeks he had developed a weeping eczematous rash in flexural areas, which was treated with topical emollients and low potency corticosteroids.

His mother said that he had been irritable and difficult to feed from the age of 2 months but had received the standard immunisation schedule; he had reacted to the vaccination at 4 months with a fever and a purpuric rash which had subsided over a period of 4 days. Since his first chest infection, he had suffered from episodes of coughing and wheezing. Some developmental delay had also been diagnosed at a recent child surveillance clinic. Oscar was not yet sitting unaided and had failed the distraction test for hearing. There was no family history of atopy or recurrent infections. Oscar's sister, aged 18 months, was fit and well and had no history of developmental delay.

On examination Oscar was on the 3rd centile for weight and height. He was drowsy throughout the interview and was clearly unwell. His nappy contained loose, blood stained stools. He had no dysmorphic features or evidence of jaundice but appeared pale. His forehead and maxillae were covered with a purpuric, haemorrhagic rash and flexural, exudative eczema was present.

His pulse was 145 beats/min and he had a temperature of 37.9°C. His respiratory rate was elevated at 50 breaths/min but he had no further signs of respiratory distress. Auscultation demonstrated a few diffuse crackles and inspiratory wheezes in both lung fields. A cardiovascular examination was normal with no added heart sounds. His abdomen was soft and non-tender with no palpable masses. Both testes were normal.

Oscar's right tympanic membrane was perforated and purulent fluid was present in the external auditory meatus (EAM). His pharynx and oral cavity were normal. The results of investigations are shown in *Figure 11.1*.

An underlying diagnosis of Wiskott–Aldrich syndrome was made based on immunodeficiency, thrombocytopaenia and eczema. Oscar's otitis media was treated with intravenous ceftazidime and his haematological status was monitored. He was not very anaemic and did not require red cells immediately but his thrombocytopaenia was an indication for a transfusion of fresh platelets.

QUESTIONS

1 How is Wiskott–Aldrich syndrome inherited?
2 What clinical features characterise the syndrome?
3 What treatment options are available?

Investigation	Result (normal range)
Haemoglobin (g/dl)	8.2 (13.5–18.0)
White cell count (x 10^9/l)	8.5 (6.4–11.0)
Neutrophils (x 10^9/l)	6.8 (2.0–7.5)
Eosinophils (x 10^9/l)	0.12 (0.4–0.44)
Total lymphocytes (x 10^9/l)	1.8 (2.7–5.4)
T lymphocytes (x 10^9/l)	0.8 (2.7–5.3)
B lymphocytes (x 10^9/l)	1.1 (0.6–1.4)
Platelets (x 10^9/l)	35 (150–400)
Blood film	Normocytic red cells Small platelets
Serum immunoglobulins	
IgG (g/l)	10.6 (2.4–8.8)
IgM (g/l)	0.2 (0.02–2.10)
IgE (IU/ml)	98 (0.3–20)
IgA (g/l)	0.91 (0.1–0.5)
Antibodies made in response to immunisations	
Diphtheria	Present
Tetanus	Present
Measles	Present
Rubella	Present
Haemophilus influenzae B	Absent
Antibodies to infectious agents	
Herpes simplex virus	Absent
Varicella-zoster virus	Absent
Cytomegalovirus	Absent
Epstein–Barr virus	Absent
Antibodies to ABO antigens	Below normal levels
RAST	
D. pteronyssinus	Positive
Cat	Negative
Wheat	Positive
Egg	Positive
Milk	Negative
Blood culture	Negative
Urine culture	Negative
Culture of exudate from EAM	*H. influenzae*
CSF	No sign of infection
Chest X-ray	Diffuse shadowing in both lung fields
Abdominal X-ray	Normal
Liver function tests	
Serum albumin (g/l)	35 (35–50)
Alkaline phosphatase (IU/l)	395 (30–300)
Aspartate transaminase (IU/ml)	32 (5–35)
Serum bilirubin (μmol/l)	9 (3–17)
Prothrombin time (secs)	12.1 (10–14)
Activated partial thromboplastin time (secs)	38.9 (35–45)
Maternal chromosome analysis	Non-random X-chromosome inactivation

Fig. 11.1 Results of investigations.

■ **CASE 11**   pp. 289, 291

ANSWERS

1   How is Wiskott–Aldrich syndrome inherited?

Wiskott–Aldrich syndrome (WAS) is an X-linked recessive immunodeficiency disorder. Initial studies aimed at finding the molecular defect in WAS focused on a cell surface glycoprotein CD43 (sialophorin). CD43 is a 400 amino acid integral transmembrane glycoprotein of molecular weight 115 kDa expressed on thymocytes, T and B lymphocytes, monocytes, granulocytes and platelets. It has signal transduction capability and therefore plays a role in lymphocyte activation. It also putatively binds to ICAM-1, a cell adhesion molecule. The finding that lymphocytes from WAS patients have absent or abnormal CD43 suggested that a defect in activation or adhesion may cause WAS. A direct role for CD43 was excluded however when its gene was localised to chromosome 16.

More recent linkage studies have localised the WAS gene to the Xp11.22-p11.23 region of the X chromosome. The previously unrecognised gene, named Wiskott–Aldrich syndrome protein (WASP), is expressed in cell lines of lymphocytic and megakaryocytic origin. WASP encodes a 501 amino acid protein of unknown function which is proline-, glycine- and leucine-rich. Lymphoblasts from WAS subjects do not appear to express the gene. Deletions and point mutations in WASP have been identified in unrelated patients. It appears that the majority of mutations occur in the four exons at the N-terminus of the gene. The location of the mutations does not appear to correlate with the phenotype. Female carriers of the WAS gene preferentially inactivate the affected X-chromosome, a marker which can be used to aid diagnosis. Since the gene has been sequenced, genetic probes can be developed to allow definitive diagnosis. WASP is known to bind to several signalling proteins belonging to the lec family of tyrosine kinases (which includes btk). WASP also appears to act as an actin-depolymerising agent protein. It can be hypothesised that WASP has a role in signal tansduction to organise cortical actin filaments, and therefore cytoskeletal structure.

2   What clinical features characterise the syndrome?

WAS was first described by Wiskott in 1937. He reported a family in which three male children suffered from repeated infections, thrombocytopaenia and severe flexural eczema. Aldrich characterised the X-linked recessive nature of the disease in 1954. The disorder is rare with four new cases per million live births. Affected subjects usually present in infancy with episodes of bleeding, most frequently bloody diarrhoea. Epistaxis, petechiae and intracranial bleeding are also common. The thrombocytopaenia is worsened by infections, which may cause melaena, haematuria or haematemesis.

Episodes of infection begin at 4–6 months of age. Bacterial infections may be caused by both Gram-positive and negative organisms, presenting as pneumonia, otitis media and sinusitis. Viral infections include cytomegalovirus, varicella-zoster and herpes simplex which may become widespread and fatal. Eczema also starts at 4–6 months and is indistinguishable from atopic dermatitis. There is an increased risk of lymphoreticular malignancy in WAS subjects, usually non-Hodgkin's and Hodgkin's lymphoma or leukaemia.

The platelets are reduced in number and in size with an average count of approximately $20 \times 10^9/l$. Patients are often anaemic and have a prolonged bleeding time. Lymphocyte counts are normal at birth but diminish with age, with the decrease largely in the $CD4^+$ population. Serum IgG is usually normal with decreased levels of IgM and increased IgA and IgE. Antibody production to polysaccharide antigens (e.g. *Haemophilus influenzae B* (HiB) vaccine) are absent and iso-haemagglutinins (anti-ABO antibodies) are reduced or absent.

3   What treatment options are available?

Supportive management includes the prompt diagnosis and treatment of infections and the use of platelet transfusions to ameliorate any thrombocytopaenia. Topical and oral steroids may be used to control the eczematous lesions despite coexistent immunodeficiency. Splenectomy increases both platelet numbers and size and decreases the number of bleeding episodes. The increased risk of infection associated with splenectomy (see Case 1) can be combated with the use of prophylactic antibiotics or intravenous gammaglobulin.

HLA matched bone marrow transplantation completely reverses the thrombocytopaenia, immunodeficiency and eczema and is the treatment of choice when a donor is available. Analysis of a long series of WAS patients calculated the median survival as 5.7 years. The use of bone marrow transplantation has undoubtedly increased this figure with several recipients known to have survived into adulthood. Common causes of death are infection (59%), haemorrhage (27%) and malignancy (5%). The isolation of WASP suggests that gene therapy may become a viable option in the future.

■ CASE 12

Mr Doyle, a 52-year-old record producer, was seen in Accident & Emergency with a 1-week history of worsening shortness of breath accompanied by an unproductive cough, mild chest pain, fever and malaise. He had no previous history of angina and was a life long nonsmoker. Medical history included gonorrhoea and genital herpes within the past 3 years. Over the past 2 months he had suffered from persistent diarrhoea accompanied by a weight loss of 9 kg from an initial baseline of 68 kg. For the past week he had complained of pain on swallowing which he attributed to a sore throat. He had lived with his male partner with whom he had been having unprotected intercourse for several years. There was no history of intravenous drug use.

On examination, Mr Doyle was underweight and mildly febrile. He had no oedema but lymph nodes were palpable in his cervical, axillary and inguinal regions. Plaques of *Candida albicans* were visible on his pharyngeal wall. He had a pulse of 102 beats/min and a respiratory rate of 25/min at rest. Chest expansion was reduced and there were mild diffuse crackles across both lung fields. His optic fundi were normal. The results of investigations are shown in *Figure 12.1*.

Because of his sexual history Mr Doyle was counselled regarding a human immunodeficiency virus (HIV) test and consented. An enzyme-linked immunosorbent assay (ELISA) was positive for anti-HIV antibodies and a polymerase chain reaction (PCR) test directly demonstrated HIV-1. A clear diagnosis of acquired immunodeficiency syndrome (AIDS) was made and Mr Doyle's *Pneumocystis carinii* pneumonia was treated with oxygen by mask and parenteral co-trimoxazole. He was discharged on prophylactic oral co-trimoxazole.

Within 3 months he was seen again in Accident & Emergency with blurred vision and 'flashing lights' in his eyes. Fundoscopy demonstrated cytomegalovirus (CMV) retinitis which was treated with parenteral ganciclovir. A CD4 T-lymphocyte count at this time was $0.04 \times 10^9/l$. Whilst receiving treatment Mr Doyle became increasingly unwell and drifted into a semi-conscious state. The results of investigations are shown in *Figure 12.2*

A diagnosis of cryptococcal meningitis was made and parenteral amphotericin was started. Mr Doyle failed to respond to treatment and died shortly afterwards. At post mortem, *P. carinii* were isolated from his lungs, and evidence of early cerebral lymphoma was noted.

QUESTIONS

1 What diagnostic tests are available for HIV infection?
2 Which of these tests should be used if HIV infection is suspected in a mother and her child, infected vertically?
3 What serological and cellular indices can be used to monitor the course of HIV infection?

Investigation	Result *(normal range)*
Haemoglobin *(g/dl)*	12.8 *(13.5–18.0)*
Platelet count *(x 10⁹/l)*	128 *(150–400)*
White cell count *(x 10⁹/l)*	6.2 *(4.0–11.0)*
Neutrophils *(x 10⁹/l)*	5.4 *(2.0–7.5)*
Eosinophils *(x 10⁹/l)*	0.24 *(0.4–0.44)*
Total lymphocytes *(x 10⁹/l)*	0.75 *(1.6–3.5)*
T lymphocytes CD4⁺ *(x 10⁹/l)*	0.12 *(0.7–1.1)*
CD8⁺ *(x 10⁹/l)*	0.42 *(0.5–0.9)*
B lymphocytes *(x 10⁹/l)*	0.11 *(0.2–0.5)*
Arterial blood gases	
PaO₂ *(kPa)*	7.8 *(>10.6)*
PaCO₂ *(kPa)*	5.52 *(4.7–6.0)*
pH	7.39 *(7.35–7.45)*
HCO₃⁻	25.6
Base excess	-0.9
ECG	Normal
Chest X-ray	Bilateral diffuse interstitial shadowing
Bronchoscopy with bronchoalveolar lavage	Positive for *Pneumocystis carinii*

Fig. 12.1 Results of investigations.

Investigation	Result *(normal range)*
Haemoglobin *(g/dl)*	10.4 *(13.5–18.0)*
Platelet count *(x 10⁹/l)*	104 *(150–400)*
White cell count *(x 10⁹/l)*	4.1 *(4.0–11.0)*
Neutrophils *(x 10⁹/l)*	4.2 *(2.0–7.5)*
Eosinophils *(x 10⁹/l)*	0.24 *(0.4–0.44)*
Total lymphocytes *(x 10⁹/l)*	0.62 *(1.6–3.5)*
T lymphocytes CD4⁺ *(x 10⁹/l)*	0.03 *(0.7–1.1)*
CD8⁺ *(x 10⁹/l)*	0.40 *(0.5–0.9)*
B lymphocytes *(x 10⁹/l)*	0.09 *(0.2–0.5)*
Chest X-ray	Minimal areas of diffuse shadowing
Blood culture	Negative
Blood glucose *(mmol/l)*	7.6 *(<10.0)*
CSF from lumbar puncture	
Appearance	Turbid
White cells *(polymorphs/mm³)*	2500
Protein *(g/l)*	4.2 *(0.15–0.45)*
Glucose *(mmol/l)*	4.5 *(>60% blood glucose)*
Indian ink stain	Positive for cryptococcus

Fig. 12.2 Results of investigations.

■ **CASE 12**   pp. 291–292, Chapter 16

ANSWERS

1   What diagnostic tests are available for HIV infection?

Approximately 95% of HIV-positive individuals seroconvert within 3 months of infection. ELISAs for antibodies to gp41, an HIV surface glycoprotein, and p24, a core protein, are the most widely used to detect HIV infection. Confirmation is obtained by Western blot analysis to decrease the rate of false positive results. The Centre for Disease Control recommends that the blot should be positive for 2 of the p24, gp41 and gp120/160 markers (gp160 is the precursor form of gp41 and gp120, the envelope protein). ELISAs for p24 antigen can also be used although the false negative rate is higher.

The polymerase chain reaction (PCR) is a technique for amplifying specific sequences of DNA or RNA to produce quantities that are readily detectable. The test in the context of HIV is highly sensitive and specific but is more costly than ELISA techniques.

2   Which of these tests should be used if HIV infection is suspected in a mother and her child, infected vertically?

The mother's serological state should be tested by ELISA and confirmed by Western blot if positive.

Around 20–30% of infants born to HIV positive mothers are infected with the virus. Transmission can occur *in utero* or very rarely by breast feeding. Diagnosis presents a problem because maternal IgG specific for HIV antigens crosses the placenta and can be detected in the infant even if it has not become infected.

The presence of HIV specific antibodies of IgA and IgM classes in the infant should imply infection because they do not cross the placenta. Current tests lack sensitivity and remain in development. The method most widely used in the UK and USA is PCR which demonstrates the virus directly. Below the age of 1 month PCR may be negative in infected children. It has been shown that, in many children, HIV is sequestered into regional lymph nodes at this age. After establishing infection at these sites a viraemia follows.

3   What serological and cellular indices can be used to monitor the course of HIV infection?

Figure 12.3 shows the change in a variety of indices of HIV infection over time. Acute seroconversion causes an infectious mononucleosis-like illness in up to 50% of those infected with HIV. Common symptoms are fever, lymphadenopathy, pharyngitis, rashes and myalgia. At this point there is a drop in the CD4 (and also CD8) lymphocyte count and a rise in plasma viraemia and p24 antigen concentration. Antibodies to HIV surface glycoproteins gp120 and gp41 are produced from approximately 6 weeks after infection and are initially of the IgM class. IgG antibodies of the same specificities follow the IgM response and persist during the latent phase. Viraemia and p24 antigenaemia are generally low during this period. Disease progression is heralded by a declining CD4 lymphocyte count and a rise in plasma viraemia. Clinically, CD4 counts have become a widely used index of progression. Plasma viraemia is the most accurate measure of disease progression, and is becoming a more commonly used method. Appendix 11 shows the major clinical complications at different CD4 counts.

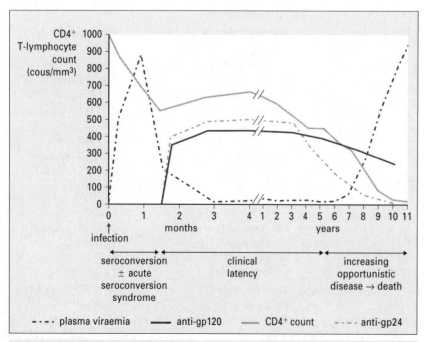

Fig. 12.3 A typical course of HIV infection.

■ CASE 13

Mr Middleton, a 33-year-old accountant, was seen in Accident & Emergency in an acute confusional state. His brother, when contacted by phone, was able to give a limited history. Mr Middleton had become increasingly unwell over the preceding year. He had lost almost 13 kg in weight, and had a 6-month history of profuse, watery and bloody diarrhoea. The diarrhoea had been previously investigated, and was believed to have been caused by ulcerative colitis. He had also consulted a dermatologist for a persistent rash on his back. No further history was available, although the brother was sure that Mr Middleton was a practising homosexual.

On examination, Mr Middleton was disoriented in time, space and person. He was frightened and uncooperative, and had been incontinent of urine and faeces. Clinically, he was dehydrated and pale and had cold, cyanosed peripheries. Some small left sided cervical lymph nodes were palpable and he had a temperature of 35.5°C. His chest was clear except for a few crackles at both bases, and he had a respiratory rate of 12/min. He was tachycardic with a pulse of 115 beats/min regular and had a blood pressure of 128/82 mmHg. His abdomen was difficult to examine, but there were no obvious abnormalities. A central nervous system examination was similarly difficult, but he was moving all four limbs without difficulty. Mr Middleton's mouth showed evidence of candidiasis and oral hairy leukoplakia. There was evidence of fungal infection beneath the finger- and toenails. Results of investigations are shown in *Figure 13.1*.

A provisional diagnosis of HIV disease was made, and further investigations performed to elucidate the cause of the acute confusional state. Medazolam, 5 mg, was administered to render the patient cooperative for radiology and lumbar puncture. The results of further investigations are shown in *Figure 13.2*.

Mr Middleton was started on 2 g of cefotaxime intravenously three times daily, and 200 mg of oral fluconazole daily. Over the following 24 hours his condition deteriorated and there was increasing confusion. He developed marked shortness of breath and a dry cough. Oxygen saturations dropped to 95% on air, and a repeat chest X-ray showed worsening lung infiltrates. Oral cotrimoxazole three times daily was started for presumed *Pneumocytis carinii* pneumonia. He remained confused, with a strong element of mania, which required chlorpromazine and procyclidine therapy. As he improved, further screening tests were performed to check for exposure to other pathogens. He was negative for CMV IgM, hepatitis B and C viruses, TPHA, RPR and toxoplasma serology. His CD4 count was 28.

QUESTIONS

1 What therapeutic options are available to manage HIV disease progression?
2 Which agents could be used for:
  a) A patient with seroconversion illness?
  b) A patient with established HIV disease?
  c) An individual who has sustained a needlestick injury from a HIV positive subject?
  d) A pregnant HIV positive patient?
3 What are the causes of diarrhoea in HIV positive patients?

Investigation	Result (normal range)
Haemoglobin (g/dl)	11.0 (13.5–18.0)
White cell count (x 10⁹/l)	5.7 (4.0–11.0)
Neutrophil count (x 10⁹/l)	3.7 (2.0–7.5)
Lymphocyte count (x 10⁹/l)	1.3 (1.6–3.5)
Eosinophil count (x 10⁹/l)	0.0 (0.4–0.44)
MCV (fl)	83.5
Platelet count (x 10⁹/l)	197 (150–400)
Serum	
Sodium (mmol/l)	144 (134–145)
Potassium (mmol/l)	4.2 (3.5–5.0)
Creatinine (mmol/l)	45 (70–105)
Urea (µmol/l)	7.2 (2.5–6.7)
Liver function tests (mmol/l)	Normal
Glucose (mmol/l)	4.2
C reactive protein (mg/l)	17 (<5)
Paracetamol	Not detected
Salicylate	Not detected
Oxygen saturation	98% on air

Fig. 13.1 Results of investigations.

Investigation	Result (normal range)
CT scan of brain	No mass lesions, no enhancing lesions, mild involutional change, no evidence of raised intracranial pressure
Chest X-ray	Bilateral patchy mid/upper zone consolidation
CSF from lumbar puncture	
Appearance	Clear
White cells (polymorphs/mm³)	<1
Red cells (/mm³)	<1
Protein (g/l)	0.23 (0.15–0.45)
Glucose (mmol/l)	1.7 (>60% blood glucose)
Lactate (mmol/l)	Negative
Gram stain	Negative
Indian ink stain	Negative
Cryptococcal antigen	Negative
HIV ELISA	Positive

Fig. 13.2 Results of further investigations.

■ **CASE 13**   pp. 296–299

ANSWERS

1 What therapeutic options are available to manage HIV disease progression?

The aim of intervention with therapeutic agents in HIV disease is to impair viral replication and hence prevent increasing viraemia, which is a marker of disease progression. Until recently, monotherapy with nucleoside analogues was the only available option to prevent progression of HIV disease. These agents inhibit HIV reverse transcriptase by terminating the development of the viral RNA chain. Examples include zidovudine (AZT), didanosine (ddI), zalcitabine (ddC), stavudine (d4T) and lamivudine (3TC). All have potential side effects including bone marrow suppression (AZT) and peripheral neuropathy (ddI, ddC, d4T, 3TC). Two new classes of drugs are the protease inhibitors, which prevent viral maturation (e.g. ritonavir, indinavir, saqunavir), and the non-nucleoside reverse transcriptase inhibitors.

Recent attention has focused on combinations of these drugs. There is now good evidence to suggest that double therapy with either two nucleoside analogues, or one nucleoside analogue plus a protease inhibitor, is more effective than monotherapy. A wide selection of trials has shown that almost all combinations appear effective in reducing disease progression as monitored by CD4 counts. Furthermore, it appears that triple-therapy combinations are more effective than double therapy.

2 Which agents could be used for:

a) A patient with a seroconversion illness?

If a patient presents with the early stages of HIV disease, zidovudine for 6 months has been shown to delay disease progression.

b) A patient with established HIV disease?

Triple therapy is now widely used in patients with newly diagnosed, but advanced HIV infection. Therapy should be commenced before the CD4 count drops below 350/ml. The actual agents used vary between centres, but clearly compliance and drug interactions are important issues.

c) A person who has sustained a needlestick injury from an HIV positive subject?

Data from the USA, UK and France have shown that the transmission rate of HIV from needlestick injuries can be reduced by 80% if zidovudine is administered for 3–4 weeks after the incident.

d) A pregnant HIV positive mother?

Treatment of the mother before and during birth, in combination with treatment of the newborn child using zidovudine, reduces the risk of transmission to the child by two-thirds.

3 What are the causes of diarrhoeal illnesses in HIV positive subjects?

Diarrhoea is one of the most common complaints in HIV infected subjects, with the majority experiencing the symptom at some point in the course of the disease. Protracted diarrhoeal illnesses are often troublesome and difficult to treat. A wide range of bacteria, viruses and protozoa may cause diarrhoea, some of which are also common in seronegative subjects.

Bacteria

Campylobacter, Salmonella and *Shigella* species are commonly implicated. *Campylobacter jejuni* infection often causes watery diarrhoea associated with colicky abdominal pain. *Salmonella* and *Shigella* can produce invasive disease resulting in bloody diarrhoea.

Bacteraemia (salmonellosis) is, as one would expect, a more common complication.

Mycobacterium avium intracellulare (MAI), which can affect almost any organ system, can cause a diarrhoeal illness in HIV infected individuals. MAI invades the intestinal mucosa to produce white plaques that are visible on colonoscopy.

Viruses

HIV itself may be responsible for a proportion of diarrhoeal illnesses. Cytomegalovirus can often produce a severe colitis, often with bloody stools. As in other forms of colitis, colonic dilatation can occur, and this may present with an acute abdomen.

Protozoa

Cryptosporidium, an intracellular parasite found in sheep and cattle, is the commonest cause of diarrhoea in HIV. The stools are usually profuse and watery, and malabsorption commonly occurs with a protracted illness. The oocytes of the protozoa can be identified in the stool using a Ziehl–Neelsen stain.

CASE 14

Justin was born at 41 weeks by forceps delivery after an uneventful pregnancy. At birth he weighed 3.7 kg and had no physical abnormalities. Aged 13 months he developed bilateral swellings in his inguinal region, which became increasingly inflamed. Within several days the swellings began to discharge purulent fluid through multiple sinuses. On examination he was febrile and irritable and had reduced weight and head circumference for his age. Culture of the fluid revealed *Staphylococcus aureus* as the cause of the infection, and he was treated with flucloxacillin.

Aged 15 months Justin was seen in Accident & Emergency with a high fever, irritability, malaise and failure to feed. On examination he was clearly unwell and had a temperature of 39.0°C. He was below the 3rd centile for weight and height for his age. His spleen and liver were enlarged and tender and he had lymphadenopathy in the inguinal and cervical regions. Examination of his left leg revealed a tender, red and fluctuant swelling of the knee joint. His mother recalled him receiving the standard immunisation schedule without any adverse reactions. The results of investigations are shown in *Figure 14.1*.

A diagnosis of acute osteomyelitis with pyogenic arthritis was made and Justin was started on parenteral flucloxacillin and gentamicin. His hepatosplenomegaly was further investigated with a CT scan which demonstrated multiple radio-opaque lesions within the liver. Histology of a CT-guided liver biopsy showed microabscesses and non-suppurative giant-cell granulomas.

While convalescing in hospital Justin developed a red fluctuant swelling on his thoracic wall which required surgical drainage and further antibiotics. The causal organism was identified as *Pseudomonas aeruginosa*. The results of investigations during this infection are shown in *Figure 14.2*.

A diagnosis of chronic granulomatous disease was made and Justin remained in hospital to receive further antibiotic therapy. Prophylactic anti-bacterial and anti-fungal agents were also prescribed. Within the next year he was readmitted twice for recurrent staphylococcal abscesses, which were treated aggressively with prolonged courses of parenteral high dose antibiotics and surgical drainage.

QUESTIONS

1 What is the pathogenesis of chronic granulomatous disease (CGD) and how is it inherited?
2 What is the basis of the diagnostic tests for CGD?
3 How should CGD patients be managed?

Investigation	Result *(normal range)*
Haemoglobin *(g/dl)*	12.4 *(13.5–18.0)*
White cell count *(x 10^9/l)*	25.6 *(6.8–10.0)*
Serum	
Sodium *(mmol/l)*	141 *(134–145)*
Potassium *(mmol/l)*	4.3 *(3.5–5.0)*
Chloride *(mmol/l)*	104 *(95–105)*
Creatinine *(µmol/l)*	97 *(70–150)*
Blood culture	Negative
Chest X-ray	Normal
Abdominal X-ray	Diffuse hepatic shadowing
X-ray of knee joints	Involucrum and sequestrum of the distal left femur with a purulent effusion of the left knee

Fig. 14.1 Results of investigations.

Investigation	Result *(normal range)*
White cell count *(x 10^9/l)*	26.3 *(6.8–10.0)*
Neutrophils *(x 10^9/l)*	21.2 *(2.0–7.5)*
Eosinophils *(x 10^9/l)*	0.88 *(0.4–0.44)*
Total lymphocytes *(x 10^9/l)*	4.1 *(2.0–4.1)*
T lymphocytes *(x 10^9/l)*	2.1 *(2.7–5.3)*
B lymphocytes *(x 10^9/l)*	0.1 *(0.6–1.4)*
Serum immunoglobulins	
IgG *(g/l)*	17.2 *(3.0–15.8)*
IgG1 *(g/l)*	10.6 *(1.5–9.8)*
IgG2 *(g/l)*	4.2 *(0.3–3.9)*
IgG3 *(g/l)*	1.1 *(0.1–0.8)*
IgG4 *(g/l)*	0.71 *(0.05–0.65)*
IgM *(g/l)*	2.7 *(0.4–2.2)*
IgE *(IU/ml)*	11 *(3–22)*
IgA *(g/l)*	1.7 *(0.15–1.3)*
Serum	
C3 *(g/l)*	1.98 *(0.75–1.65)*
C4 *(g/l)*	0.80 *(0.20–0.65)*
Antibodies made to immunisations	All present at normal levels
Nitroblue tetrazolium reduction test	Absent dye reduction
In vitro incubation of leucocytes with *S. aureus*	Decreased bacterial killing compared with controls

Fig. 14.2 Results of further investigations.

■ CASE 14   pp. 229–239, 294

ANSWERS

1 What is the pathogenesis of chronic granulomatous disease (CGD) and how is it inherited?

Chronic granulomatous disease is a term which covers a group of rare inherited disorders involving the respiratory burst in phagocytic cells (macrophages/monocytes and polymorphs). The incidence is between 1:250 000 and 1:1 000 000 births/year.

The respiratory burst is characterised by the *de novo* production of superoxide anions by the reaction:

$$NADPH + 2O_2 \longrightarrow NADP^+ + 2O_2^- + H^+$$

The superoxide O_2^- reacts rapidly to produce hydroxyl free radicals, hydrogen peroxide and hypochlorous acid, which all have bacteriocidal activity. The reaction is catalysed by an NADPH-oxidase found in phagocytes (*Fig. 14.3*). This enzyme consists of at least five subunits which are assembled on activation of the cell by phagocytosis or chemotactic peptides. The activation process involves the phosphorylation of p47-*phox* and the migration of p47- and p67-*phox* from the cytosol to the cell membrane where they become associated with cytochrome b 558. With the subunits assembled the reaction depicted above is catalysed and the respiratory burst proceeds.

CGD is caused by inherited mutations within the genes encoding the cytochrome subunits (*Fig. 14.4*). Phagocytosis occurs normally in affected patients but pathogenic organisms persist within the cell due to an absent respiratory burst. Their presence stimulates granuloma formation whose mass effect may cause symptoms.

Common infections in these patients cause pneumonia, suppurative lymphadenitis, liver abscess, osteomyelitis and septicaemia. The organisms most frequently responsible are *Staphylococcus aureus*, *Escherichia coli*, *Klebsiella*, *Proteus*, *Salmonella*, *Aspergillus* and *Candida* species.

2 What is the basis of the diagnostic tests for CGD?

The nitroblue tetrazolium (NBT) test is a simple screening test for CGD. The yellow dye is reduced to blue crystals by the phagocytes if they have an intact respiratory burst. Patients with CGD are therefore NBT negative. Reduced bacterial killing is also a feature of CGD and can be assessed by the incubation of the patient's phagocytes with bacteria.

3 How should CGD patients be managed?

The life threatening nature of infections in CGD patients warrants the use of anti-microbial prophylaxis. Co-trimoxazole (trimethoprim and sulphamethoxazole) is widely used because it has intracellular killing activity and is active against staphylococcal and Gram-negative bacteria. *Aspergillus* species are also a common cause of morbidity and mortality in CGD and has prompted the use of prophylactic itraconazole. Intradermal injections of interferon-gamma (IFNγ) are also beneficial. The addition of IFNγ to phagocytes from CGD patients *in vitro* induces a partial correction of the diminished superoxide formation.

Acute infections should be treated vigorously with drugs which penetrate phagocytes. Surgery may be necessary to relieve pressure from granulomata (e.g. in the gut where they may cause obstruction) or to drain abscesses.

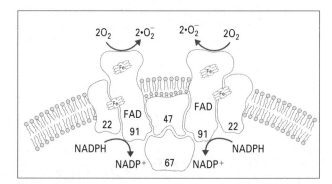

Fig. 14.3 Schematic model of phagocyte NADPH oxidase.

	Protein				
	Cytochrome b 558 α-subunit p22-*phox*	**Cytochrome b 558 β-subunit gp 91-*phox***	**p47-*phox***	**p67-*phox***	**rac 1/rac 2**
MW (kDa)	22	91	47	67	Unknown
Protein site	Integral transmembrane	Integral transmembrane	Cytosol	Cytosol	Cytosol
Gene	16q24	Xp21.1	7q11.23	1 q25	Unknown
Inheritance of defect	Autosomal recessive	X-linked recessive	Autosomal recessive	Autosomal recessive	None known
% of cases	<5%	~65%	~30%	<5%	—

Fig. 14.4 Components of NADPH-oxidase and defects in CGD.

■ CASE 15

Seventeen-year-old Angela was seen by her GP with a 1-day history of a painless, non-pruritic swelling of her left hand. On examination, the area was tense but not erythematous, hot or tender. The doctor made a diagnosis of urticaria and prescribed oral antihistamines. Within 3 days the swelling subsided.

One year later, Angela was admitted to Accident & Emergency with a 8-hour history of cramping abdominal pain, vomiting and anorexia. There was no history of haematemesis or bleeding per rectum. On examination she had a pulse rate of 98 beats/min, a blood pressure of 95/65 mmHg and a temperature of 36.8°C. Her abdomen was soft with no surgical scars. Some mild tenderness was present over her umbilical region but there was no rebound tenderness and her bowel sounds were normal. The results of investigations are shown in *Figure 15.1*.

Within 2 days, her abdominal pain and vomiting had subsided and were replaced by a brief period of diarrhoea. Surgery was considered unnecessary and she was treated with intravenous fluids and nil by mouth.

Six months later, Angela was readmitted to Accident & Emergency with worsening swelling of her lips and tongue following a dental extraction. Within an hour, laryngeal swelling precipitated respiratory obstruction which required immediate intubation. On examination she had a pulse rate of 93 beats/min, a respiratory rate of 26/min and a blood pressure of 95/65 mmHg. Her oropharynx and larynx were grossly swollen and erythematous. Results of investigations are shown in *Figure 15.2*.

A diagnosis of type I hereditary angioedema (HAE) was made based on the history and complement profile. Angela was referred to an immunologist for further evaluation and treatment.

QUESTIONS

1 What are the functions of C1 inhibitor (C1INH)?
2 What is the aetiology and pathogenesis of hereditary angioedema (HAE) and how does it compare with the acquired forms of the disease?
3 What treatments are available?

Investigation	Result *(normal range)*
Haemoglobin *(g/dl)*	13.2 *(11.5–16.0)*
White cell count *(x 10⁹/l)*	15.3 *(4.0–11.0)*
Serum	
Sodium *(mmol/l)*	140 *(134–145)*
Potassium *(mmol/l)*	4.8 *(3.5–5.0)*
Chloride *(mmol/l)*	101 *(95–105)*
Creatinine *(µmol/l)*	88 *(70–150)*
Urine microscopy	~5 white cells/ml
Culture	<10⁴ mixed organisms/ml
Pregnancy test	Negative
Plain abdominal X-ray	Enlargement of small bowel loops
Abdominal X-ray after barium meal and follow through	Thickening of the jejunal and ileal walls with evidence of mucosal oedema and narrowing of the bowel lumen

Fig. 15.1 Results of investigations.

Investigation	Result *(normal range)*
Haemoglobin *(g/dl)*	15.5 *(11.5–16.0)*
White cell count *(x 10⁹/l)*	7.4 *(4.0–11.0)*
Neutrophils *(x 10⁹/l)*	4.8 *(2.0–7.5)*
Eosinophils *(x 10⁹/l)*	0.30 *(0.4–0.44)*
Total lymphocytes *(x 10⁹/l)*	6.2 *(1.6–3.5)*
Serum immunoglobulins	
IgG *(g/l)*	12.1 *(5.4–16.1)*
IgM *(g/l)*	1.1 *(0.5–1.9)*
IgA *(g/l)*	1.4 *(0.8–2.8)*
IgE *(IU/ml)*	30 *(3–150)*
Skin prick tests to a variety of common allergens	No positive wheals
RAST for common allergens	Negative
Serum albumin *(g/l)*	38 *(35–50)*
Serum	
Sodium *(mmol/l)*	147 *(134–145)*
Potassium *(mmol/l)*	5.0 *(3.5–5.0)*
Chloride *(mmol/l)*	107 *(95–105)*
Creatinine *(µmol/l)*	105 *(70–150)*
Serum complement	
C1q *(mg/l)*	150 *(100–250)*
C2 *(mg/l)*	5 *(10–30)*
C3 *(g/l)*	1.25 *(0.75–1.65)*
C4 *(g/l)*	0.09 *(0.2–0.65)*
C1 inhibitor (C1INH)	
Antigenic	<30%
Functional	<30%
Chest X-ray	Normal

Fig. 15.2 Results of further investigations.

ANSWERS

1 What are the functions of C1 inhibitor (C1INH)?

C1INH is a 478 residue single-chain polypeptide member of the serine protease (Serpin) superfamily coded on chromosome 11. It is primarily synthesised by the liver but other cells, notably peripheral blood monocytes, also contribute. C1INH acts as an inhibitor for a variety of proteases by structurally mimicking their substrates (see Appendix 6).

2 What is the aetiology and pathogenesis of hereditary angioedema (HAE) and how does it compare with the acquired forms of the disease?

Angioedema is characterised clinically by acute swelling of subcutaneous or submucosal tissues with no pruritus. Common sites are the extremities and the gastrointestinal tract. In addition, two-thirds of patients develop orofacial or laryngeal lesions which may cause respiratory distress or asphyxia. The aetiology of angioedema is multifactorial with C1 inhibitor deficiencies constituting a minority. C1INH deficiency can be classified as hereditary or acquired (*Fig. 15.3*).

Hereditary angioedema is caused by a deficiency of C1INH. Two forms of HAE exist, both transmitted as an autosomal dominant trait. Heterozygotes have disease, as the single normal gene is able to maintain serum levels at only 5–30% of normal. In HAE I the transcription or translation of C1INH is impaired, leading to decreased serum levels of normal protease, whilst in HAE II the serum level is normal but the protease lacks functionality.

Acquired angioedema also exists in two forms. The majority of patients with angioedema do not have a recognisable aetiology and form the idiopathic group. It has recently been recognised that angiotensin converting enzyme (ACE) inhibitors, used in the treatment of hypertension and cardiac failure, precipitate angioedema in approximately 0.1% of patients taking the drug. A possible explanation lies in the ability of ACE to convert bradykinin to inactive peptides (see Appendix 6), although it remains unclear why only a proportion of patients are susceptible.

In all cases a decrease in the functional activity of C1INH to less than 35% of normal is associated with a risk of an acute attack of angioedema. In addition to this biochemical predisposition, triggering events such as endotracheal tubes or dental manipulations are important in the majority of patients. It is believed that endothelial trauma leads to the activation of factor XII (Hageman factor) and the triggering of the coagulation and complement pathways. The paucity of C1INH allows the accumulation of active components from these pathways which may in turn produce angioedema. It remains unclear whether bradykinin or C2 kinin is the major contributor to this process.

3 What treatments are available?

In an acute attack involving the larynx or facial region maintenance of the airway is critical. Intravenous fluids should be used to correct hypovolaemia and appropriate pain relief provided. C1INH concentrate can be administered and has been shown to alleviate attacks. Fresh frozen plasma, which contains C1INH, is a cheaper and readily available alternative.

Preventative therapy for HAE includes the use of attenuated androgens such as danazol which directly increase the transcription, translation and secretion of C1INH. Antifibrinolytic agents such as tranexamic acid which inhibit plasmin activity may also be useful.

In acquired angioedema (AAE) I an underlying cause should be vigorously sought and maintenance treatment given as for HAE. Such treatments are of dubious value in AAE II where immunosuppression and plasmapheresis are used.

Type	%	Defect	Causal factors	C1INH (antigenic levels)	C1INH (functional levels)	C1	C3	C4
Hereditary angioedema type I (HAE I)	>80%	Impaired mRNA transcription or translation	Base deletions	<30%	<30%	N	N	⬇
Hereditary angioedema type II (HAE II)	~15%	Production of non-functional C1INH	Base deletions	≥100%	<30%	N	N	⬇
Acquired angioedema type I (AAE I)	Rare	Excess activation of C1 leading to excess consumption	B-cell lymphoproliferative disorders with autoantibody production, e.g. chronic lymphocytic leukaemia	<30%	<20%	<30%	N	⬇
Acquired angioedema type II (AAE II)	Rare	Autoantibodies stop binding, allowing C1s to cleave C1INH to inactive form	None known, not associated with malignancy	70–100%	<10%	⬇	N	⬇

Fig. 15.3 Aetiology and serological features of angioedema.

CASE 16

Sixty-two-year-old Mrs Young was stung by a bee from a hive in her back garden. Harvesting the honey had left her with several stings during the course of the summer. Several minutes after the recent sting she complained of an itching sensation in her hands, feet and groin accompanied by cramping abdominal pain. Shortly afterwards she felt faint and acutely short of breath. Moments later she collapsed and lost consciousness. Her husband, a doctor, noticed that her breathing was rapid and wheezy and that she had swollen eyelids and lips. She was pale and had patchy erythema across her neck and arms.

On examination her apex beat could be felt but her radial pulse was weak. Her husband immediately administered 0.5 ml of 1/1000 adrenaline intramuscularly and 10 mg of chlorpheniramine (an H_1-receptor antihistamine) intravenously with 100 mg of hydrocortisone. She regained consciousness and her respiratory rate dropped. By the following day she had recovered completely. Results of investigations at this time are shown in *Figure 16.1*.

Mrs Young had no history of adverse reactions to bee venom, foods or antibiotics. In addition there was no history of asthma, allergic rhinitis, food allergy or atopic dermatitis. A diagnosis of anaphylactic shock due to bee venom sensitivity was made based on the history and investigations and a decision taken to commence desensitisation therapy.

She was made aware of the possible risk of the procedure and consented to it. She was injected subcutaneously with gradually increasing doses of bee venom, the procedures being performed in hospital with access to resuscitation apparatus. No further allergic reactions occurred and she was maintained on a dose of bee venom at 1-month intervals for the next 2 years. She was stung by a bee the following summer and had no adverse reaction.

QUESTIONS

1 What mechanisms are involved in anaphylaxis?
2 What are the clinical features and management of acute anaphylaxis?
3 How may such sensitivity be detected and what can be done to desensitise patients?

Investigation	Result (normal range)
Haemoglobin (g/dl)	14.2 (11.5–16.0)
White cell count (x 10⁹/l)	7.5 (4.0–11.0)
Neutrophils (x 10⁹/l)	4.4 (2.0–7.5)
Eosinophils (x 10⁹/l)	0.40 (0.4–0.44)
Total lymphocytes (x 10⁹/l)	2.4 (1.6–3.5)
Platelet count (x 10⁹/l)	296 (150–400)
Serum immunoglobulins	
IgG (g/l)	10.2 (5.4–16.1)
IgM (g/l)	0.9 (0.5–1.9)
IgA (g/l)	2.1 (0.8–2.8)
IgE (IU/ml)	320 (3–150)
RAST	
Bee venom	Class 4
Wasp venom	Class 0
Skin prick tests	Grade (0–5)
Bee venom (10 µg/ml)	3+

Fig. 16.1 Results of investigations.

■ **CASE 16**   p. 302

ANSWERS

1 What mechanisms are involved in anaphylaxis?

Traditionally, the term anaphylaxis has been used to describe a systemic clinical syndrome caused by IgE mediated degranulation of mast cells and basophils. Susceptible individuals exposed to a sensitising antigen produce specific IgE antibodies which bind to high affinity IgE receptors (FcεRI) found on mast cells and basophils. The receptor binds the Fc portion of the antibody leaving the Fab binding sites available to interact with antigen. The avidity of this Fc binding reaction is high and therefore the dissociation of IgE from the receptors is slow, with a long half-life. On subsequent exposure, the antigen is bound by the IgE receptor complexes, which causes receptor mediated activation of the cells with release of preformed and *de novo* synthesised mediators (see Appendix 7). Degranulation is rapid and is completed within 30 minutes. These mediators, released on a large scale, are responsible for the clinical manifestations of anaphylaxis.

The IgE mediated mechanism of mast cell degranulation has been implicated in the pathogenesis of anaphylaxis triggered by a variety of agents. These include antibiotics (e.g. penicillins, cephalosporins), foods (e.g. milk, nuts, shellfish), foreign proteins (e.g. insulin, bee venom, latex) and pharmacological agents (e.g. streptokinase, vaccines). The patient may or may not have a history of atopy. Indeed, natural allergen exposure in atopics is a rare cause of anaphylaxis.

Mast cell degranulation can occur by IgE independent pathways. Prior exposure is not a prerequisite as specific IgE antibodies are not involved. Three putative mechanisms of anaphylactoid reactions are given below:

- Blood, blood products and immunoglobulins can cause an anaphylactoid reaction. The suggested mechanism is the formation of immune complexes with subsequent complement activation and production of C3a and C5a. Both of these complement components (anaphylatoxins) are capable of degranulating mast cells directly. In addition both components increase vasopermeability and may induce hypotension. Mellitin, a major component of venom, is able to activate the alternative pathway of complement and also produce an anaphylactoid reaction through anaphylatoxins.

- Certain therapeutic and diagnostic agents such as opiates, ACTH, muscle relaxants and contrast media are also capable of directly causing mast cell degranulation and anaphylaxis.

- Five to ten percent of asthmatic subjects produce a reaction to non-steroidal anti-inflammatory drugs (NSAIDs), such as aspirin or indomethacin. Symptoms commonly include bronchospasm, rhinorrhoea and, rarely, vascular collapse. The ability of these agents to cause anaphylaxis appears to correlate with their effectiveness in inhibiting prostaglandin synthesis. The mechanism of this sensitivity is unknown but may involve mast cell degranulation in some patients.

2 What are the clinical features and management of acute anaphylaxis?

There is a great variation in the timing and nature of anaphylactic symptoms. The onset is usually within seconds or minutes of exposure although delays of an hour have been reported. The following are common presentations which may occur singly or in combination:

- Cutaneous: erythema, pruritus of hands, feet and abdomen, urticaria, angioedema.
- Respiratory: laryngeal oedema causing hoarseness which may progress to asphyxia, bronchoconstriction causing wheezing, rhinorrhoea.
- Cardiovascular: hypotension, arrhythmias, tachycardia, vascular collapse.
- Gastrointestinal: cramping abdominal pain, nausea, vomiting, diarrhoea.

The majority of cases of anaphylactic reactions are not fatal. It has been estimated that 1–2% of courses of penicillin therapy are complicated by systemic reactions but only 10% of these are serious. In the USA some 400–800 people die annually from penicillin anaphylaxis with a similar figure for contrast media. Seventy percent of deaths result from respiratory complications (laryngeal oedema and/or bronchospasm) with 25% resulting from cardiovascular dysfunction.

Prompt treatment of anaphylaxis is essential as death may occur rapidly. The patient is placed in the recovery position, oxygen is given by mask and 0.5–1.0 ml of adrenaline is injected intramuscularly. This has the effect of raising the blood pressure, relaxing bronchial smooth muscle and preventing further mediator release. Intravenous antihistamines (e.g. 10 mg of chlorpheniramine) can be useful as histamine can cause vasodilatation, cardiac arrhythmias and bronchospasm. Corticosteroids (e.g. 100 mg of hydrocortisone) intravenously may help to reduce any late phase response (see Case 18).

3 How may such sensitivity be detected and what can be done to desensitise patients?

The first step is to obtain a thorough history of previous adverse reactions. The timing and nature of such reactions should be noted. Skin prick testing with insect venom is a fast and sensitive method of detecting anti-venom IgE. Radioallergosorbent tests can detect venom specific IgE, but are positive in only 80% of those with significant reactions to venom skin prick tests.

Immunotherapy is best reserved for those with life threatening systemic reactions to insect venom. The patient is given increasing subcutaneous dosages and is then given a monthly maintenance dose of 100 μg. The clinical protection rate is in the order of 98% for both adults and children.

■ CASE 17

Mr Nez was rather surprised to find after so many years of feeling well that at the age of 28 he had begun to get a blocked nose. All his friends and business colleagues commented that he appeared to have a continuous cold! In fact he did have problems with recurrent sinusitis, consisting of face pain and a purulent discharge from his nose. His GP prescribed several courses of antibiotics, which relieved the symptoms for a time. He was perhaps slightly better during the summer months.

After another attack of sinusitis he went to an ENT surgeon. Investigations at that time are shown in *Figure 17.1*. A diagnosis of chronic maxillary sinusitis was made and the ENT surgeon recommended an antral puncture and washout.

At operation, the sinuses were washed out and then drained. A submucous diathermy was also performed. His post-operative course was uneventful. He was told by the surgeon that he would be very much better after the surgery.

After an interval of only 3 months, the original symptoms had returned, including a further attack of sinusitis for which he had another course of antibiotics. He was then sent to an allergist for evaluation. His nose was congested and the turbinates were covered in excess secretions. There was no evidence of infection. The results of the further investigations are shown in *Figure 17.2*.

He was started on a local nasal corticosteroid aerosol and at the same time specific immunotherapy for his house-dust mite allergy. He did extremely well and had no further symptoms.

QUESTIONS

1 What are the results of allergen exposure in the nose?
2 What genetic factors are involved in atopy?
3 What is the role of the eosinophil in allergic rhinitis?
4 What techniques are available for hyposensitisation?

Investigation	Result *(normal range)*
Haemoglobin *(g/dl)*	14.2 *(13.5–18.0)*
White cell count *(x 10⁹/l)*	10.8 *(4.0–11.0)*
Serum	
Sodium *(mmol/l)*	138 *(134–145)*
Potassium *(mmol/l)*	4.2 *(3.5–5.0)*
Chloride *(mmol/l)*	100 *(95–105)*
Urea *(mmol/l)*	3.6 *(2.5–6.7)*
Serum immunoglobulins	
IgG *(g/l)*	10.5 *(5.4–16.1)*
IgM *(g/l)*	1.2 *(0.5–1.9)*
IgA *(g/l)*	2.1 *(0.8–2.8)*
Sinus X-ray	Thickened mucosa with a fluid level in the left maxillary antrum

Fig. 17.1 Results of investigations.

Investigation	Result *(normal range)*
Total IgE *(IU/ml)*	540 *(3–150)*
Skin prick tests to	
House dust mite	Positive
Grass pollen	Positive
RAST	Grade *(0–5)*
House dust mite	4+
Grass pollen	2+
Mucociliary clearance	Normal
Chest X-ray	Normal

Fig. 17.2 Results of further investigations.

■ **CASE 17**　　pp. 302, 308, 305

ANSWERS

1 What are the results of allergen exposure in the nose?

The nasal mucosa is lined by mast cells which express the high affinity receptor for IgE (FcεRI). The number of mast cells increases during the season due to an increased migration of cells from the lamina propria into the epithelium as well as actual proliferation of the mast cells within the nasal mucosa. Following allergen challenge or exposure during the season, there is an immediate release of preformed mediators such as histamine with itching, sneezing and rhinorrhoea as well as the synthesis of newly formed mediators from arachidonic acid. The late phase reaction occurs 5–8 hours after the exposure and consists of a recurrence of symptoms, with more nasal obstruction than sneezing.

Using nasal lavage, histamine, PGD_2, and kinins can be found in the early phase, all being characteristic of mediators derived from mast cells. During the late phase reaction, a similar profile of mediators is found, with the exception of PGD_2, which is absent. This implicates the basophil as responsible for at least part of the late phase reaction.

Sodium cromoglycate will block the immediate reaction as well as the late phase response. Corticosteroids will block only the late phase response. Both rhinitis and asthma respond to corticosteroids, suggesting that the late phase reaction is the more important from the clinical point of view.

2 What genetic factors are involved in atopy?

Allergic reactions involve interactions between the make up of the individual and factors in the environment.

Genetic responses are best seen where the allergen is completely characterised and is of low molecular weight. Ragweed contains at least 55 allergens of which only half are important clinically. The major allergen Amb a 1, has a molecular weight of 35 kDa, whereas Amb a 5 is the smallest yet identified at 4.5 kDa. There is a strong association of an Amb a 5 response with the HLA DR2*1500 genotype governing both the IgE and IgG responses. Rye grass allergy (Lol P 1) is also associated with HLA DR2. Heritability of serum IgE levels has also been shown in family and twin studies but the location of the gene has not yet been defined.

These factors are relatively simple compared with the actual manifestation of allergic (atopic) symptoms in a patient. Taking a very simplistic view, Cookson and colleagues defined an atopic patient as having an elevated IgE, and specific IgE as measured by RAST or skin tests. Their studies suggested a link between atopy and locus 11q13, and that the atopy gene was inherited preferentially from the maternal side. Recent data from Marsh suggested that the atopic link is with genes controlling IL-4.

3 What is the role of the eosinophil in allergic rhinitis?

The changes to the nasal mucosa immediately after challenge with allergen show the result of mast cell degranulation with very little cell accumulation. If the same area is lavaged 48 hours later, there is a marked increase in eosinophils as well as other cells. The higher the allergen dose, the more eosinophils are seen as well as their products such as major basic protein (MBP). IL-5 is the predominant cytokine seen in the lavage fluid. This is an eosinophil chemoattractant as well as contributing to the longer life of the cell.

The ligand which allows the eosinophil to bind to endothelium is VCAM-1: this binds to the cell adhesion molecule VLA-4. Using allergic sheep, it is possible to show that pretreating them with a monoclonal antibody against VLA-4 significantly reduces the late phase reaction following bronchial provocation with allergen but has no effect on the immediate reaction. These observations clearly show the role of the eosinophil in allergic reactions in the lung and nose.

4 What techniques are available for hyposensitisation?

The classic method was pioneered by Noon and Freeman in 1911 and consisted of giving incremental amounts of the relevant allergen by subcutaneous injection until an arbitrary top dose was reached. They checked the response to treatment by performing quantitative ocular challenges with the allergen to assess the change in sensitivity. Since that time, incremental immunotherapy (IT) has been the mainstay of treatment. There are other techniques using low dose allergen that have been shown to be effective and safe. The actual mechanism(s) by which IT leads to clinical improvement has not yet been elucidated.

With the advent of molecular cloning techniques, recombinant allergens are now available. This has been useful as it has shown that many allergens cross react and the number needed for the diagnosis and even treatment of Type 1 hypersensitivity may be limited.

There are three main approaches to IT:

- Interfering with the allergen–IgE interaction. This is the concept of blocking antibodies whether induced in the patient or derived from recombinant Fabs in human or mouse.
- Prevention of allergen induced mast cell/basophil degranulation. Cross linking of IgE on the effector cell is the key event leading to degranulation. Local application of hapten could theoretically saturate the free IgE Fabs, thus blocking the cross-linking process and the resulting degranulation.
- Modulation of IgE by IT. There is a trend for the level of specific IgE to fall after IT but in many cases the allergen extract is crude. Isolation of the T cell epitope of the allergen, totally devoid of any IgE binding would have several advantages. It would be completely safe with no danger of anaphylactic side effects. It might also induce T-cell tolerance to that specific allergen.

An exciting area is that of expressing allergens in live vaccine strains. These may induce strong T-helper cell (TH) 1 responses and thus be useful as therapeutic agents for atopy.

■ CASE 18

Nine-year-old Jennifer was seen by her GP with a 4-month history of coughing, wheezy breathing and insomnia. The symptoms had become progressively worse over this period which spanned August to November. Her mother reported that Jennifer's cough was often worse at night, and that leaving for school on cold winter mornings also exacerbated her symptoms. She had been unable to participate in school games for several weeks due to breathlessness on exertion. Recently, she had become extremely breathless and wheezy after helping her mother clean the house.

Jennifer was born at term after an uneventful pregnancy and had no previous history of prolonged respiratory tract infections. Her mother had opted for bottle rather than breast feeding from birth. Childhood illnesses had included measles, mumps and atopic eczema, which had proved refractory to topical emollient and corticosteroid therapy. Seasonal allergic rhinitis linked to pollen exposure had started at 5 years of age and was being treated with oral antihistamines. There was no history of food allergy. Jennifer's mother had also had atopic eczema up to adolescence and suffered from seasonal allergic rhinitis.

The family home was carpeted throughout and Jennifer's room had curtains and a large collection of soft toys. The pet cat, which had been a resident for five years, had access to all rooms of the house. None of the family members smoked.

On examination Jennifer was on the 50th centile for height and weight. She had no finger clubbing, tachycardia or fever. She was not tachypnoeic at rest, had good chest expansion, and resonant lung fields to percussion. On auscultation she had a mild expiratory wheeze in both lung fields. Her nasal turbinates were mildly inflamed and covered with a mucous exudate. Her throat and tympanic membranes were normal and there was no evidence of allergic conjunctivitis. A cardiovascular examination showed no abnormality. A dry, scaly, eczematous rash was present in both elbow and knee flexures. The results of investigations are shown in *Figure 18.1*.

A diagnosis of allergic (extrinsic) asthma was made. Her doctor recommended regular vacuuming of the house to reduce dust levels. He also advised that the curtains in Jennifer's room should be cleaned frequently and that her soft toys should be placed in the freezer overnight on a regular basis to eliminate dust mites. Further allergen avoidance recommendations included the use of plastic mattress and pillow covers and an air filter. The doctor also suggested removal of the pet cat. A compromise in the face of stiff opposition was to prevent the cat entering Jennifer's bedroom.

An inhaled dose of salbutamol, a β_2 adrenoceptor agonist, produced an increase in the peak expiratory flow rate and resolved Jennifer's cough. She was provided with a metered dose inhaler of salbutamol and was advised to use it as needed for symptomatic relief. A further inhaler containing sodium cromoglycate was prescribed for regular use on a three times daily basis. Her doctor also provided a peak flow meter and asked Jennifer's mother to keep a daily diary of measurements to aid treatment of her asthma. A self-management plan gave the family guidance in modifying medication when symptoms became severe and provided a way of recognising severe exacerbations requiring medical attention.

The combination of the two drugs was sufficient to control her asthma, which resolved by the age of 22.

QUESTIONS

1 How can allergic asthma be defined, and what aetiological factors have been identified?
2 What pathological findings are present in the lungs of a patient with allergic asthma?
3 What is the mechanism of allergic asthma?

Investigation	Result (normal range)
Haemoglobin (g/dl)	12.5 (11.5–16.0)
White cell count (x 10⁹/l)	13.7 (4.0–11.0)
Neutrophils (x 10⁹/l)	6.8 (2.0–7.5)
Eosinophils (x 10⁹/l)	1.23 (0.4–0.44)
Total lymphocytes (x 10⁹/l)	2.5 (2.0–4.1)
Serum immunoglobulins	
IgG (g/l)	12.3 (5.4–16.1)
IgM (g/l)	1.2 (0.5–1.8)
IgA (g/l)	2.2 (0.5–2.5)
IgE (IU/ml)	325 (3–150)
Peak expiratory flow rate	Below normal for height and age
Lung function tests	
FEV1:FVC ratio	68%
Chest X-ray	Normal
Skin prick tests	Grade (0–5)
D. pteronyssinus	3+
Cat	3+
Dog	0
Cockroach	0
Mixed grasses	3+
Foods	All negative
Sputum examination	Large quantities of green mucoid plugs and eosinophils

Fig. 18.1 Results of investigations.

■ **CASE 18**   pp. 302, 308, 310–315

ANSWERS

1 How can allergic asthma be defined, and what aetiological factors have been identified?

Asthma can be defined as an inflammatory condition of the lungs characterised by reversible paroxysmal airways obstruction. Common presenting symptoms are a cough, shortness of breath and wheezing. The cough is often worse at night and may be exacerbated by exercise. Epidemiological studies have charted a rising prevalence of asthma worldwide, with the UK figure currently more than 5% in children and 2% in adults. Around 2000 people die annually from acute severe asthma in the UK. Asthma is a multifactorial disease dependent on several genetic and environmental factors.

Asthma has a familial incidence and surveys suggest that if one parent has asthma the chance of their offspring developing the disease is around 1 in 6. The inheritance of a complex allergic disease, such as asthma, cannot be explained by a single gene inheritance.

Environmental factors are also important in the development of asthma. Exposure to inhalant allergens in infancy is correlated with the development of allergic disease. Parental smoking and viral respiratory tract infections also increase the incidence of asthma. The month of birth and its relation to seasonal allergen exposure and subsequent atopy may also be of importance.

2 What pathological findings are present in the lungs of a patient with allergic asthma?

In chronic asthma, the bronchial blood vessels are dilated and there is an inflammatory exudate within the interstitium. The connective tissue and smooth muscle compartments increase in size and there is an enlarged volume of epithelial cells. The basement membrane is thickened by an increased deposition of type IV collagen. The mucous secreting glands are enlarged by goblet cell metaplasia and there is sloughing of epithelial cells into the bronchial lumen.

The lumen often contains an inflammatory exudate referred to as a 'mucous plug'. In fact the majority of the exudate consists of fluid derived from blood vessels, proteins, sloughed epithelium and migrating inflammatory cells. The eosinophil and mast cell count in the exudate is often high with many cells in a necrotic state.

The increase in size of bronchial wall components and the presence of an exudate in the lumen produce minimal reductions in the calibre of the airways. However, computer models have demonstrated that a contraction of 40% by the bronchial smooth muscle superimposed on these chronic pathological changes is sufficient to occlude the bronchial lumen completely.

3 What is the mechanism of allergic asthma?

Acute exacerbations of allergic asthma causing bronchospasm are initiated by mast cell degranulation. Samples obtained from the airways of asthmatics by bronchoalveolar lavage (BAL) show 3–5 fold increases in mast cells compared with normal subjects.

In susceptible individuals the mast cells are primed with specific IgE antibodies, and following cross-linking by allergen, a variety of preformed and *de novo* synthesised mediators are released. These cause bronchoconstriction, vasodilation of pulmonary vessels and increased mucus production. BAL studies in asthmatics have shown 5–15 fold increases in mast cell mediators compared with normal subjects.

Eosinophils are also important mediators of airway inflammation. The full thickness of the bronchial wall is infiltrated with eosinophils, many of which are degranulated. Eosinophils are capable of binding IgE via high and low affinity IgE receptors. Cross-linking these receptors with allergen through bound IgE causes release of eosinophil granule proteins which can damage respiratory epithelium, degranulate mast cells and cause contraction of bronchial smooth muscle.

The production of IgE antibodies to common inhalant allergens, for example house dust mite and cat, is promoted by the predominant TH2 subset in the bronchial inflammatory infiltrate. These lymphocytes produce IL-4 which is responsible for inducing B cells to switch antibody production to the IgE class and has an autocrine effect on mast cells. IL-3, IL-5 and GM–CSF, also produced by TH2 cells, have eosinophil chemotactic and activation properties.

Following an acute attack, many patients with allergic asthma have a late phase response which usually starts at 5–8 hours after the initial exposure, peaks at 12 hours and subsides by 36 hours. Histologically this is characterised by an influx of neutrophils, eosinophils and lymphocytes into the epithelium and submucosa. These cells are recruited into the lung by mast cell mediators released during the early response.

Clinically, patients with early and late phase responses have two corresponding troughs in their peak flow measurements.

A model for the pathogenesis of allergic asthma begins with a genetically susceptible individual exposed to allergen, probably within the first 4 years of life. The allergens are processed by antigen presenting cells (APCs) and presented to specific T cells. These cells differentiate into TH2 clones which promote IgE production and the eosinophilic response. Re-exposure to the allergen in synergy with other factors such as viral respiratory tract infections, exercise and exposure to tobacco smoke, triggers acute and chronic inflammatory responses in the airways manifested as reversible airways obstruction.

■ CASE 19

When James was 9 months old, he began to scratch his skin at night. He had an itchy rash on his face, rather vesicular in type, which became infected and he needed a course of antibiotics. When he was 18 months old, he had scratches on his wrists, elbows and behind his knees, which became thickened and dry. He also had cracks behind his ears.

His nose had been rather blocked and runny over the past few months and his mother thought that he was occasionally wheezy at night but did not associate the wheezing with anything in particular. He had never had nappy rash and his mother thought that the itching and scratching must be due to the new washing powder that she had bought. Even when she changed back to the old one, the rash continued to get worse.

One day at breakfast, James decided to try some of his brother's peanut butter sandwich, or at least to rub some of it on his face. Within minutes he had a red face with swelling of his cheeks and eyes, he began to scream, and his lips started to swell. His mother took him straight to the GP and fortunately by the time he got there the swelling had started to settle down.

When the doctor examined him he found a lively baby with typical atopic eczema. He had a generally dry skin, marked flexural lesions and a rather blocked crusty nose. Where James had smeared the peanut butter on his face was red and inflamed and the doctor said that it would be dry and scaly by the next day – looking much more like acute eczema then.

The results of the investigations done at that stage are shown in *Figure 19.1*.

In view of the skin tests, environmental precautions were taken in the following way. The family cat was banished from sleeping on James' bed during the day and had to live in the outhouse. His mother changed his pillows to ones made of artificial fibre and covered his mattress with a special washable cover. The carpets in his room were removed as were the velvet curtains. His soft toys were put in the deep freeze from time to time and then in the tumble dryer to kill the house dust mites.

His eczema cleared to a great extent when he stopped eating foods containing milk. He had never really liked cooked eggs by themselves but was able to eat cake. His mother was warned never to give him peanuts. She was also advised to have an adrenaline syringe at home and to get James a Medicalert bracelet labelled with his diagnosis, including 'peanut anaphylaxis'.

QUESTIONS

1 What are the changes seen in the skin in atopic eczema?
2 Do airborne allergens play a part in inflammation of the skin?
3 What immunological abnormalities are found in atopic eczema?
4 What are the genetic factors involved in atopic eczema?

Investigation	Result (normal range)
Haemoglobin (g/dl)	13.8 (13.5–18.0)
White cell count (x 10⁹/l)	9.8 (6.8–10.0)
Eosinophils (x 10⁹/l)	1.2 (0.4–0.44)
Lymphocytes (x 10⁹/l)	4.2 (2.0–4.1)
Neutrophils (x 10⁹/l)	4.5 (2.0–7.5)
Serum IgE (IU/ml)	940 (3–22)
RAST	Grade (0–5)
Grass	3+
House dust mite	4+
Milk	2+
Egg	2+
Peanut	4+
Cat	3+
Skin prick tests to:	
Grass	Positive
House dust mite	Positive
Cat	Positive
Egg, milk	Positive
Cockroach	Positive
No skin test with peanut allergen	

Fig. 19.1 Results of investigations.

■ **CASE 19** pp. 302, 310–311

ANSWERS

1 What are the changes seen in the skin in atopic eczema?
It is only relatively recently that strict criteria were laid down for the diagnosis of atopic eczema. There are four basic features:

- Itching. It is considered by some to be a hallmark of atopic eczema, as bronchial hyperreactivity is considered characteristic of bronchial asthma.
- Typical morphology with lichenification in adults and involvement of the face in children.
- Chronic or relapsing disease.
- Personal or family history of atopy.

The skin is typically dry with many scratch marks. The dryness may be explained by increased epidermal water loss perhaps associated with an abnormal fatty acid profile in the skin and reduced δ-6 desaturase activity. There is a marked cellular infiltrate in the skin which resembles an allergic contact dermatitis. Lymphocytes are mainly CD4+ and the majority express HLA-DR as a sign of activation. There is an increased expression of the low affinity IgE receptor (FcεRII, CD23) on Langerhans' cells in the skin, which also express the high affinity receptor (FcεRI). Keratinocytes in lesional skin show surface adhesion molecules ICAM-1. There are increased numbers of mast cells, some of which show signs of degranulation. Eosinophil derived products such as major basic protein (MBP) can also be seen in the skin using histochemical techniques.

The cytokine profiles in the skin suggest activation of TH2 cells predominantly but in chronic lesions there is also evidence for IFNγ suggesting TH1 involvement.

2 Do airborne allergens play a part in inflammation of the skin?
Exacerbations of skin lesions can be elicited by inhalation of pollen or house dust. There is also evidence that allergen can penetrate through the skin.

Positive reactions similar to those found in contact dermatitis have been shown using house dust mite applied to the skin as patch tests. A reddening and eczematous reaction is seen under the patch when examined after 1–2 days. The severity of the local response can parallel the concentration of circulating specific IgE to house dust mite.

In the lesions in the skin following the patch test, Langerhans' cells showing both allergen and IgE were found in the epidermis in the first few hours and after 24–48 hours were found in the dermis. Eosinophils can also be found in the skin 6 hours after application of the patch test.

These data support the concept that eczema is, in part, an IgE-mediated contact hypersensitivity. Further evidence for this view comes from the observations that identical antigen specific T-cell clones could be obtained from patch test lesions and lesional skin biopsies from the same patient.

Children play on carpets and also sleep in beds where substantial amounts of house dust mite allergen are found. It is likely that large amounts of house dust mite may be scratched into the skin during exacerbations of the disease and contribute to the immunological response. Allergen elimination measures should be considered for all children with atopic eczema.

3 What immunological abnormalities are found in atopic eczema?
There is considerable evidence for immunological abnormalities in atopic eczema. These can be characterised by:

- High IgE levels. These are much higher than those seen in any other atopic disease. Some patients have levels of IgE in the range of 30 000 IU/ml where the normal level is 100 IU/ml. This alone suggests an abnormal T-cell control of B-cell function. This can be shown by culturing atopic eczema peripheral blood mononuclear with normal or atopic T cells. The former can suppress IgE production *in vitro* whereas the latter are less effective. This shows a functional lack of suppressor activity.
- Impaired T-cell function. Defective cell mediated immunity is seen in up to 80% of atopic eczema patients as measured by recall skin testing for delayed type hypersensitivity or by patch testing for contact allergy. Patients also have an unusual susceptibility to vaccinia and severe skin infections with herpes simplex. A variety of techniques can show that the T-cell ratios in patients are also abnormal. Early studies showed a reduction in CD8+ cells with an increase in CD4+ cells. These changes were not seen in patients with allergic rhinitis or asthma.
- TH1/TH2 lymphocytes. When T-cell clones are made from patients with atopic disorders, there is a significant shift to TH2 cells. In atopic patients who are sensitive to both *D. pteronyssinus* and tetanus toxoid, IL-4 is produced in response to the house dust mite stimulus whereas IFNγ is induced by the tetanus antigen. The role of IL-13 in the induction of an IgE response remains to be elucidated.

4 What are the genetic factors involved in atopic eczema?
There is a clear family history of atopy in patients who have atopic eczema with a significant increase in the number of relatives suffering from asthma, hay fever, urticaria and food allergy. The most compelling evidence for genetic factors is from the study of twins. If genetic factors were the only cause of eczema, then identical (monozygotic) twins would always have the same disease, i.e. be 100% concordant. Nonidentical twins (dizygotic) would show the same incidence as would siblings in the same family. The data show that indeed monozygotic twins are more concordant for atopic eczema (risk 0.74) compared with dizygotic twins (risk 0.23). This shows that genetic influences play a decisive role in the development of the skin disease. However, there are cases where there is a marked discordance in monozygotic twins. In these cases, the environment presumably plays the decisive role.

■ CASE 20

Forty-seven-year-old Mr Brewer went to his GP complaining of some wheezing in his chest. He had recently had an episode of bronchitis that consisted of some shortness of breath and a cough with sputum, which contained mucous plugs. His doctor did find some prolongation of expiration and his peak expiratory flow rate was 434 l/min, which was 70% of that predicted for his height and age. His FEV1 was also reduced (*Fig. 20.1*). The doctor agreed that he had some asthma but also thought that he had bronchitis as well. He was given a course of antibiotics which did not help his symptoms. He was then given a salbutamol inhaler and an inhaled corticosteroid which did help.

Some weeks later Mr Brewer returned to the doctor with increased breathlessness in spite of the treatment. He had been gardening and moving a little compost but did not really feel that this small amount of gardening alone had aggravated matters. His asthma was definitely worse and it was felt necessary to give him some oral corticosteroid treatment which in 10 days had produced a dramatic improvement in his health. The tablets were tapered off and nothing more was heard from Mr Brewer for 6 months.

He reappeared with yet another cough, slight fever and definite wheezing. This time he was referred to a chest physician for further evaluation.

When he was examined, he had signs of asthma and his lung function tests showed evidence of both restrictive and obstructive patterns. The results of the other investigations are shown in *Figure 20.2*.

He was thought to have extrinsic asthma and given a further course of oral corticosteroids, which resolved the symptoms. His cough started again and it was thought wise to organise a bronchoscopy, which showed plugging of the right mid-zone bronchus with a yellow mucoid plug; this was aspirated.

Culture of the plug showed growth of *Aspergillus fumigatus*. His serum was then assayed for precipitating antibodies to *A. fumigatus*, and it was strongly positive. A diagnosis was then made of allergic bronchopulmonary aspergillosis (ABPA).

QUESTIONS

1 What are the *Aspergillus*-related lung diseases?
2 What are the diagnostic criteria and staging for ABPA?
3 What is known about the pathogenesis of ABPA?
4 What are the causes of bronchopulmonary eosinophilia?

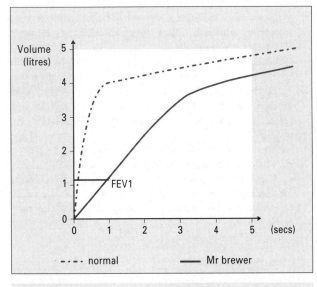

Fig. 20.1 Pulmonary function tests. The FEV1 is low in the patient compared with a matched control, indicating the presence of airways obstruction.

Investigation	Result *(normal range)*
Haemoglobin *(g/l)*	13.5 *(13.5–18.0)*
White cell count *(x 10⁹/l)*	9.2 *(4.0–11.0)*
Neutrophils *(x 10⁹/l)*	7.2 *(2.0–7.5)*
Eosinophils *(x 10⁹/l)*	1.65 *(0.4–0.44)*
Lymphocytes *(x 10⁹/l)*	3.4 *(1.6–3.5)*
Serum IgE *(IU/ml)*	664 *(3–150)*
RAST	Grade *(0–5)*
Grass	4+
House dust mite	4+
A. fumigatus	4+
Skin prick tests	
Grass	Positive
House dust mite	Positive
Cat	Positive
A. fumigatus	Positive
Precipitins	
A. fumigatus	Positive

Fig. 20.2 Results of investigations.

■ **CASE 20**   pp. 229–240, 329–330

ANSWERS

1 What are the *Aspergillus*-related lung diseases?

It is likely that an atopic who makes IgE following exposure to low dose environmental allergens, will respond to *A. fumigatus* with asthma. This is the case with Mr Brewer as he already had positive skin tests to common inhalant allergens.

In a non-atopic patient, the *Aspergillus* may lead to invasive aspergillosis, especially in patients with a compromised immune system. Neutropenia is a susceptibility factor for the invasion. Invasion of bronchial walls by *Aspergillus* does not occur in patients with ABPA.

Where there is a pre-existing area of bronchiectasis, the fungus may grow in the cavity and produce a fungus ball – an aspergilloma.

As with many occupational lung diseases, a typical Type III hypersensitivity may result producing a form of extrinsic allergic alveolitis as seen in Malt Worker's Lung. Inhalation of *Aspergillus* spores is a hazard of paper mill workers who also develop an hypersensitivity pneumonitis.

There is a rare form of necrotising pneumonia which occurs in immunosuppressed patients due to invasion of *Aspergillus*.

2 What are the diagnostic criteria and staging for ABPA?

To make a diagnosis of ABPA it is necessary to show specific reactivity of the patient to *A. fumigatus*. This is done by skin testing and serology.

The diagnostic features of the syndrome are asthma, chest X-ray infiltrates, positive immediate skin tests to *A. fumigatus*, elevated total IgE, precipitating antibodies to *A. fumigatus*, peripheral blood eosinophilia and elevated specific IgE and IgG to *A. fumigatus*.

Diagnostic difficulties arise when either the serology is negative or the symptoms do not clearly fit into only the diagnostic category of ABPA.

Stage I represents an acute onset, as in Mr Brewer, with positive serology, eosinophilia and infiltrates on chest X-ray.

Stage II in remission may show only a slightly elevated total IgE.

Stage III is an exacerbation where all the previous symptoms and signs of Stage I are repeated.

Stage IV represents a more chronic state where the asthma can be controlled only by long term corticosteroid therapy.

Stage V is that of lung fibrosis which is the presentation in a small group of patients. Their serology may be only marginally positive.

3 What is known about the pathogenesis of ABPA?

The serology of ABPA shows the presence of both IgG and IgE antibodies to *A. fumigatus*. A classical Type I hypersensitivity reaction to inhaled spores would produce an immediate asthmatic response. Evidence from bronchial provocation studies confirms this. However, following bronchial provocation with *A. fumigatus* allergen, there is not only an immediate fall in lung function indices but also a late fall, 5–12 hours after the challenge, lasting for a further 12–24 hours. This late phase reaction is also seen in patients who have classical Type I reactions and in that situation is due to lymphokine and mediator production leading to cell infiltration into the bronchial mucosa. These patients do not have precipitating antibodies.

Patients with EAA, for example, Farmer's Lung, do have precipitating antibodies (IgG) and this leads to local immune complex formation and fixation of complement.

Dual cutaneous reactions on skin testing are also seen providing a parallel to the reactions in the lung, i.e. a Type I skin reaction followed by an Arthus reaction 5–12 hours later.

Recent research has shown that T-cell lines from patients with ABPA are stimulated by the purified antigen Asp fI (an 18 kDa protein purified from whole extracts of *A. fumigatus*). The T cells that react have the profile of Th2 cells in producing IL-4. A role for IL-5 in the eosinophilia is expected. In animal models of ABPA, anti IL-5 inhibits the eosinophilia, confirming the role of that cytokine.

4 What are the causes of bronchopulmonary eosinophilia?

There are two main categories of patients with bronchopulmonary eosinophilia. ABPA distinguishes those patients with eosinophilia and asthma, the other category are patients who present with pneumonia and an eosinophilia. Parasites such as nematodes and microfilariae, and drugs such as busulphan, can lead to the pneumonia and eosinophilia. *A. fumigatus* can produce both asthma and pneumonia. There are other occupational causes such as epoxy resins, adverse reactions to L-tryptophan and the so-called allergic vasculitides, such as the Churg–Strauss syndrome.

Gleich and colleagues have focused on the stimuli for the eosinophilia and the mechanisms for the longevity of the cell.

Eosinophil proteins and eosinophil survival activity were much enhanced in BAL taken at 48 hours after challenge with antigen. The eosinophil survival activity was completely neutralised by anti IL-5 monoclonal antibody in most of the patients. A combination of anti IL-5 and anti GM–CSF was even more effective in neutralising the effect.

These data suggest that IL-5 is the predominant cytokine for eosinophil activity and it may well play a key role in airway inflammation where the eosinophilia is such a characteristic feature.

CASE 21

Ten-year-old Simon was seen by his doctor with a 3-week history of polyuria, excessive thirst and a weight loss of 2 kg. His mother noted that he had been sleeping excessively and that during the day he seemed lethargic. He also complained of some blurring of vision which had interfered with his school work.

Simon was born at 39 weeks following an uneventful pregnancy. Childhood illnesses included measles and mumps, which resolved without incident. He had received the standard immunisation schedule and suffered from no other major illnesses. His brother aged 7 years was fit and well but there was a family history of thyroiditis and pernicious anaemia.

On examination Simon was underweight for his height and age. Respiratory, cardiovascular, and abdominal examinations were all normal. His optic fundi were normal and there was no evidence of skin infections. His tongue and lips were dry and he appeared dehydrated. The results of investigations are shown in *Figure 21.1*.

A diagnosis of insulin-dependent diabetes mellitus (IDDM) was made. Further tests were performed to eliminate the possibility of other organ-specific autoimmune diseases in the light of an extensive family history. Thyroid function tests were normal and he was negative for anti-thyroglobulin and anti-thyroid microsomal antibodies. Serum B12 was normal and anti-intrinsic factor antibodies were negative.

Simon was referred to a dietician who advised an initial diet with excess calories to regain weight. Following this, an isocaloric diet was outlined. Carbohydrates were to contribute 50–60% of total calories with fat not exceeding 35%. Simple sugars, which produce rapid fluctuations in blood glucose, were to be replaced with complex sugars. He was also started on a regime of self-administered subcutaneous injections of insulin to normalise his blood glucose level. A mixture of short and intermediate acting insulin was prescribed to be taken twice daily, before breakfast and supper. A device for regular measurement of blood sugar was also provided. At routine follow-up Simon was coping well with the regimen and had a well controlled blood glucose level.

Investigation	Result (normal range)
Haemoglobin (g/dl)	14.2 (13.5–18.0)
White cell count (x 10⁹/l)	7.2 (4.0–11.0)
Neutrophils (x 10⁹/l)	4.6 (2.0–7.5)
Total lymphocytes (x 10⁹/l)	2.3 (2.0–4.1)
Serum	
Sodium (mmol/l)	132 (134–145)
Potassium (mmol/l)	4.5 (3.5–5.0)
Chloride (mmol/l)	93 (95–105)
Urea (mmol/l)	6.5 (2.5–6.7)
Creatinine (μmol/l)	145 (70–150)
Urine	
Glucose	+++
Ketones	+
Microscopy	~5 white cells/ml
Culture	Negative
Random blood glucose	
Test 1 (mmol/l)	12.1 (<10)
Test 2 (mmol/l)	11.7 (<10)
Anti-pancreatic islet cell antibodies	Positive by immunofluorescence

Fig. 21.1 Results of investigations.

QUESTIONS

1 What is the classification of diabetes mellitus?
2 What is the immunopathology of IDDM?
3 What genetic and environmental factors predispose to IDDM?

■ CASE 21   pp. 374–375, 135

ANSWERS

1 What is the classification of diabetes mellitus?

Diabetes mellitus (DM) may be a primary (>95%) or a secondary condition. The primary group may be further subdivided into insulin-dependent (IDDM) or type I and non insulin-dependent (NIDDM) or type II, which differ in their aetiology, pathogenesis and presentation (*Fig. 21.2*). Secondary forms of the disease can arise from other pathology (for example, pancreatitis or Cushing's syndrome) or iatrogenically.

2 What is the immunopathology of IDDM?

Type I diabetes is a disease with an underlying autoimmune aetiology. β cells of the pancreatic islets of Langerhans are selectively destroyed, although the mechanism by which this occurs is not yet fully understood. Destruction precedes the onset of overt clinical diabetes by months to years, with symptomatology commencing when the β cells have been depleted to a degree which compromises the insulin response.

Analysis of autopsy specimens from patients dying shortly after IDDM presentation reveals a lymphocytic infiltrate termed insulitis. The infiltrate is largely composed of T lymphocytes, with the CD8+ subtype predominating. Animal studies have shown that CD4+ cells are the first to infiltrate the islets with CD8+ cells migrating later. Macrophages and B cells are often also present. Significant immunoglobulin deposition is not a feature of insulitis.

A large body of evidence suggests that T cells are responsible for the destruction of β cells. For example, IDDM can be transferred to unaffected syngeneic animals by the injection of purified T cells from a non-obese diabetic mouse. The wide array of β-cell autoantibodies found in IDDM is not believed to play a significant role in islet destruction. The antibodies, which are directed against both cell surface and cytoplasmic antigens, can perhaps best be considered as markers for the disease. Insulin, proinsulin and glutamic acid decarboxylase (GAD) reactive antibodies have been demonstrated but evidence suggests that they are produced after β-cell destruction has commenced.

The β-cell antigen to which the initial autoimmune response is directed has not been characterised. Candidate antigens include GAD, insulin, heat shock protein 65 (hsp 65) and a 69 kDa protein.

3 What genetic and environmental factors predispose to IDDM?

It has long been recognised that IDDM has a familial incidence. The risk of developing IDDM to the offspring of an affected individual is around 5% with the concordance rate amongst identical twins in the order of 40%. Further familial and animal studies suggest that IDDM is a multifactorial disease influenced by environmental and polygenic components.

In man, the HLA haplotypes A1, B8, DR3 DQB1*0201 and DR4 DQB1*0302 are positively associated with IDDM. Indeed some 95% of affected individuals are HLA DR3 and/or DR4 positive. The DR2 allele has a protective effect for IDDM. The presence of an Asp residue at position 57 of the DQβ-chain also appears to be protective. Other genetic loci associated with IDDM have been identified in mice, but the search has proved elusive in man.

Multiple lines of evidence suggest environmental influences are important in the pathogenesis of IDDM. Firstly, the disease incidence varies between countries with immigrants from a low risk area moving to a higher risk area acquiring an increased risk. Secondly, the incidence in most countries is rising (e.g. Finland, where it has doubled in 15 years). Thirdly, the onset of IDDM is seasonal, peaking in the winter months and lastly, there is an absence of 100% concordance in identical twins that would be expected if the aetiology was entirely genetic.

The role of viral infections, including mumps, rubella and Coxsackie B, has long been hypothesised but it remains unclear whether the infection is a direct trigger or merely a modulator of IDDM. Recent evidence from murine models suggests that some viral infections may even be protective. It is likely therefore that the precise aetiology varies between individuals.

IDDM (type I)	NIDDM (type II)
Incidence	
1 in 400	1 in 40
Epidemiology	
Onset <40 years	Onset >40 years
M = F	M < F
Higher incidence in people of European extraction	All racial groups
Pathology	
β-cell destruction and pancreatic infiltrate of lymphocytes and macrophages	Pancreatic amyloid in 70% consisting of 37 αα protein derived from β cells
Clinical features	
Patient usually thin	Patient usually obese
Onset acute or subacute	Onset insidious
Requires insulin therapy and dietary control	Diet and/or oral hypoglycaemic agents used but insulin may be required
Liable to ketoacidotic coma	Liable to hyperosmolar non-ketotic coma

Fig. 21.2 Comparison of type I and type II insulin dependent diabetes mellitus.

■ CASE 22

Mr Edwards, a 28-year-old dry cleaner, presented in Accident & Emergency with a 2-week history of malaise, dizziness, nausea and 'puffy eyes'. He also noted that despite a normal fluid intake, he was urinating less frequently than normal. He had no haematuria and no history of a recent upper respiratory tract infection. On direct questioning he mentioned a nagging dull chest pain, which he attributed to muscular strain but this was not accompanied by a cough or haemoptysis. He smoked 20 cigarettes a day and drank socially.

On examination Mr Edwards was clinically anaemic with pale sclerae and nail beds. Diffuse oedema, especially in the lower extremities and periorbitally, was present. His blood pressure was elevated at 150/110 mmHg and his temperature was 37.8°C. His pulse rate was 87 beats/min and his jugular venous pulse could not be seen. On auscultation a few diffuse crackles could be heard in both lungs. The results of investigations are shown in *Figure 22.1*.

Mr Edwards' iron deficiency anaemia was corrected initially with a blood transfusion and followed up with intramuscular iron therapy. Within 24 hours of admission his serum urea and creatinine rose, indicating a deterioration in renal function. His urine output decreased and his proteinuria and haematuria persisted. A percutaneous renal biopsy was performed to find the cause of Mr Edwards' nephritic syndrome and renal failure. Microscopy demonstrated proliferation of glomerular endothelial and mesangial cells with a variable polymorph infiltrate. Crescent formation was also visible in part of the sample. A diagnosis of crescentic glomerulonephritis was made and further tests performed to try and find the cause (*Fig. 22.2*).

Further analysis of the biopsy specimen using fluorescence microscopy showed a linear deposition of IgG along the glomerular basement membrane. An enzyme-linked immunosorbent assay (ELISA) performed on Mr Edwards' serum demonstrated anti-glomerular basement membrane (anti-GBM) antibodies. A diagnosis of basement membrane disease (Goodpasture's syndrome) was made.

While in hospital, Mr Edwards developed frank haemoptysis and became increasingly dyspnoeic. On auscultation, his breath sounds were decreased bilaterally and he had widespread crackles. A chest X-ray showed diffuse interstitial shadowing and this, combined with a continuing low haemoglobin level, suggested lung haemorrhage. Worsening renal function and the development of lung involvement were clear indications to commence treatment. Mr Edwards was prescribed a course of corticosteroids and cyclophosphamide, which was combined with plasmapheresis to remove anti-GBM antibodies and renal dialysis to supplement poor renal function. Levels of circulating anti-GBM antibody dropped steadily over the treatment period and there was a corresponding improvement in renal function monitored by serum creatinine, and also in lung function.

While convalescing on the ward, the area around his arteriovenous shunt became infected. Concurrently his cough and haemoptysis returned and his serum urea and creatinine levels rose. Anti-GBM antibody titres were not elevated. Treatment was restarted and antibiotics were added to clear his local *Staphylococcus aureus* infection. His subsequent progress was good and he was discharged from hospital.

QUESTIONS

1 What is the aetiology of anti-glomerular basement membrane (anti-GBM) disease?
2 What is the mechanism of damage to the lung and kidney?
3 What treatment should be given?
4 Why did the skin infection at the site of the arteriovenous shunt precipitate a further episode of disease?

Investigation	Result (normal range)
Haemoglobin (g/dl)	8.2 (13.5–18.0)
White cell count (x 10⁹/l)	12.6 (4.0–11.0)
Platelet count (x 10⁹/l)	245 (150–400)
Blood film	Microcytic, hypochromic red cells
MCV	74.6
Serum	
Sodium (mmol/l)	147 (134–145)
Potassium (mmol/l)	5.1 (3.5–5.0)
Chloride (mmol/l)	107 (95–105)
Urea (mmol/l)	12.1 (2.5–6.7)
Creatinine (mmol/l)	356 (70–150)
Albumin (g/l)	27 (35–50)
Urine	
Microscopy	~5 white blood cells/ml Red blood cells ++ Granular casts
Culture	<10⁴ mixed organisms/ml
Protein	+++
Renal ultrasound scan	Both kidneys diffusely enlarged

Fig. 22.1 Results of investigations.

Investigation	Result (normal range)
Serum	
C3 (g/l)	1.21 (0.75–1.65)
C4 (g/l)	0.42 (0.20–0.65)
ANA	Negative
Anti-streptococcal antibodies	
Streptolysin O (ASO)	Negative
DNase B	Negative
Hyaluronidase	Negative

Fig. 22.2 Results of further investigations.

■ **CASE 22**   pp. 326–327, 371

ANSWERS

1 What is the aetiology of anti-glomerular basement membrane disease?

Glomerular basement membrane disease (GBM) is a rare disorder with an incidence of approximately 0.5 new cases per million population per year in the UK. It is more commonly found in men (M:F 6:1) and usually presents in the second to fifth decades of life, with the mean onset between 20 and 30 years of age.

Genetic predisposition to the disease appears to be localised to 2 separate loci. Firstly, 88% of patients with GBM disease have the HLA-DR2 haplotype compared with 30% of normal subjects. In addition, susceptibility also appears related to particular genetic variants of the immunoglobulin heavy chains. The Gm 1, 2, 21 haplotype has an increased incidence in patients with anti-GBM disease, especially if it is inherited with Gm 3, 5, 11.

Several putative triggering events have been suggested. Upper respiratory tract infections preceding the onset of disease have been identified in 20–60% of patients. The incidence of smoking amongst Goodpasture's syndrome patients is high; greater than 90% in some series. Hydrocarbon solvent exposure has also been implicated in some cases but it is unlikely to be a triggering factor in the majority.

2 What is the mechanism of damage to the lung and kidney?

GBM disease is an example of a type II hypersensitivity autoimmune disorder. Immunofluorescence microscopy demonstrates linear deposition of antibodies along the GBM or alveolar basement membrane. The antibodies are usually of the IgG class with the IgG1 subclass predominating. In addition, the C3 and C1q components of complement are often deposited. This is in contrast to the punctate deposition of immune complexes typical of Type III hypersensitivity, immune complex mediated renal disease.

The antigen to which autoantibodies are directed has recently been identified. The basement membrane is largely composed of type IV collagen with laminin, fibronectin, proteoglycans and entactin completing the structure. The primary antibody binding site is amino acid residues 198–233 found in the NC1 region of the carboxy-terminus of the 28 kD α3 chain of type IV collagen. Type IV collagen is widely distributed in human tissues, but expression of the α3 chain appears to be greatest in the GBM and alveolar basement membrane. This may provide an explanation for the restriction of anti-GBM disease to the kidney and lung.

Damage to the glomeruli and alveoli is caused by IgG mediated complement fixation. The subsequent polymorph infiltrate perpetuates the disease process.

3 What treatment should be given?

The principles of treatment are to remove the anti-GBM antibodies from the circulation and reduce their synthesis by plasmapheresis and by the use cyclophosphamide and prednisolone (*Fig. 22.3*). Patients with renal failure and oliguria require dialysis. Those who recover from the disease may have permanent renal damage warranting long term dialysis or transplantation.

4 Why did the skin infection at the site of the arteriovenous shunt precipitate a further episode of disease?

Relapses of anti-GBM mediated disease are often associated with infections of the respiratory tract, urinary tract or arteriovenous shunts used in dialysis. Anti-GBM antibody titres do not rise in the majority of those relapsing, although levels are still in excess of the normal range in all patients. Since disease activity normally correlates with antibody titre, the pathogenesis of relapse remains unclear. A possible explanation is that the threshold for renal and pulmonary damage may be lowered by ·the increased availability of acute phase reactants found during the infection.

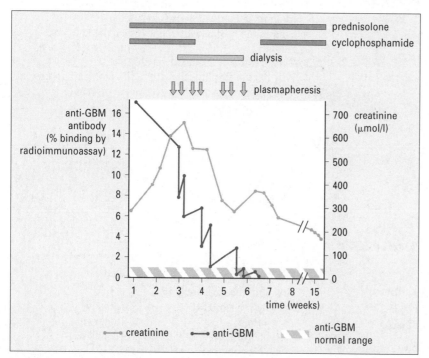

Fig. 22.3 Treatment of Goodpasture's syndrome.

CASE 23

Mrs Lake, a 30-year-old gravida 4 para 1+2, was seen at an antenatal booking clinic when 6 weeks pregnant. Her first pregnancy had been uneventful with the child, a boy, now in his teens. Her second and third pregnancies had resulted in a stillbirth at 32 weeks and a spontaneous abortion at 22 weeks, respectively. She was unaware of any reasons for the lost pregnancies and had subsequently moved from Nigeria to the UK. Medical history included uncomplicated malaria in her early twenties. She had no history of blood transfusions.

A speculum examination revealed a normal, parous cervix and there were no masses on bimanual palpation. Her blood pressure was 135/85 with the remainder of her cardiovascular and respiratory systems normal. The results of investigations, including blood grouping of the patient and her partner, are shown in *Figure 23.1*.

These results implied that the foetus was heterozygous for the D antigen and, therefore, D positive (CDe/cde). As Mrs Lake was rubella antibody negative she was advised to seek immunisation in the puerperium.

Mrs Lake's history and rhesus status were an indication for monitoring of maternal anti-D levels and foetal haemoglobin throughout the pregnancy to prevent haemolytic disease of the newborn (HDN). Serum samples taken for analysis at 3-week intervals showed a rise in maternal anti-D levels to 1.4 µg/ml at 17 weeks. Amniocentesis was performed, which yielded a sample for spectroscopic estimation of bile pigments. Severe haemolysis was demonstrated and intrauterine transfusion of the foetus was carried out using fresh (less than 7 days old), washed, CMV negative, group O, Rh D-negative blood.

Continuing risk to the child was an indication for elective caesarean section, which was performed at 34 weeks. The decision was made following assessment of foetal lung maturity by measurement of amniotic surfactant levels. A live male infant was delivered with signs of jaundice and anaemia. The results of post-partum investigations are shown in *Figure 23.2*.

Mrs Lake was given 100 µg of intramuscular anti-D antibody following delivery. Further anti-D was also administered because the Kleihauer test revealed foetal red cells in the maternal circulation at a level greater than 1 in 600. Infantile anaemia and bilirubinaemia were indications for exchange transfusion. Half a litre of Rh D-negative, CMV negative blood, ABO-matched to the child was transfused. Phototherapy was also used to degrade the bilirubin deposited in the skin. One further transfusion was required, but the child then made an uneventful recovery with no signs of kernicterus.

QUESTIONS

1 What is the mechanism of haemolytic disease of the newborn (HDN)?
2 For every 20 Rhesus-incompatible pregnancies only one or two may develop HDN. Why?
3 What is the rationale for administering anti-D antibodies to the mother?
4 Why is the incidence of ABO HDN much lower than the rate of maternofoetal ABO incompatibility?

Investigation	Result (normal range)
Haemoglobin (g/dl)	14.2 (11.5–16.0)
White cell count (x 10⁹/l)	7.6 (4.0–11.0)
Mrs Lake's blood group	A positive; Rh D-negative
Anti-D antibody	0.8 (µg/ml)
Anti-C antibody	Negative
Anti-E antibody	Negative
Anti-Kell antibody	Negative
Anti-Duffy antibody	Negative
Anti-Kidd antibody	Negative
Anti-B antibody	Present in low titre
Partner's blood group	A positive, Rh D-positive (CDe/CDe)
Sickle screening test	Negative
Rubella antibody	Negative
Urine	
Glucose	Negative
Ketones	Negative
Microscopy	~5 white cells/ml
Culture	<10⁴ mixed organisms/ml
Ultrasound scan	Normal single uterine pregnancy with visible cardiac contractions

Fig. 23.1 Results of investigations.

Investigation	Result (normal range)
Cord blood	
Haemoglobin (g/dl)	11.9 (>16.0)
Direct antiglobulin test	Positive
Blood group	Group A Rh D-positive
Infant	
Serum bilirubin (µmol/l)	325
Mother	
Kleihauer test for foetal red cells	1 in 450 (<1 in 600)

Fig. 23.2 Results of post-partum investigations.

■ CASE 23   pp. 323–324

ANSWERS

1 What is the mechanism of haemolytic disease of the newborn (HDN)?

Destruction of foetal red blood cells can occur when maternal IgG specific for red cell epitopes crosses the placenta. The cells become coated by the antibody and are destroyed by the foetal phagocytic system. In 90% of HDN cases the antibodies are directed against the Rhesus antigens. Three groups of antigens found at closely linked gene loci are included in the system. C, c, E, e and D all code for separate antigens whilst d denotes the absence of the D antigen. An individual inherits all three groups from both parents; for example cde from the mother and CDe from the father to produce the cde/CDe genotype.

In practice the majority of Rhesus incompatibilities arise from the D antigen, although anti-C, E and e antibodies may also produce HDN. More rarely, antibodies are directed against the ABO or Kell, Duffy and Kidd systems. Sensitisation to any antigen group can occur when the mother is exposed to foetal red cells following a transplacental haemorrhage, e.g. during amniocentesis or during parturition. It can also occur when a Rhesus negative mother is given Rhesus-positive blood by transfusion.

In the case of the Rhesus D antigen, the child is at risk if the mother is Rh D-negative (cde/cde) and the foetus D-positive. Initial maternal exposure to foetal red cells causes a primary IgM antibody response, which often occurs at birth. The first child is therefore not usually affected, although prolonged exposure to foetal cells during pregnancy may rarely cause HDN in a first child. Subsequent Rh D-positive children are at risk from the antibodies because they are of the IgG class and so cross the placenta freely.

The spectrum of disease caused by the incompatibility varies. In severe disease haemolysis can cause death by hydrops foetalis (severe foetal oedema) *in utero*. Moderately affected infants can be hypoxic in utero or present with symptoms of anaemia, jaundice or cardiac failure at birth. Unconjugated serum bilirubin can become deposited in the basal ganglia of the brain, leading to brain damage in a condition termed kernicterus. Affected infants often feed badly and may develop fits. Residual effects are common and include mental handicap, high-tone deafness and choreoathetosis.

Screening for HDN begins with blood grouping of the mother during early pregnancy. Rhesus negative women (15% of the population are Rhesus negative) should have anti-D antibody levels monitored throughout pregnancy. A level of 2 µg/ml, or a rapidly rising titre, are indications for amniocentesis. Patients at less than 16 weeks' gestation should have an ultrasound examination to detect foetal oedema. Blood transfusions can be provided for the foetus *in utero*, and it is usual to deliver the child electively from 32 weeks onwards if anaemia persists. Antibody titres do not correlate well with HDN severity and therefore direct foetal monitoring is more reliable. Factors believed to affect disease severity include the patient's history and the IgG subclass of the antibodies.

2 For every 20 Rhesus-incompatible pregnancies only one or two may develop HDN. Why?

It is believed that many mothers do not become sensitised to the D antigen because of maternal/foetal ABO incompatibility. If such an incompatibility exists, then foetal red cells entering the maternal circulation will be coated with antibody and destroyed before they have a chance to provoke a D-antigen specific antibody response. Anti-ABO antibodies are present despite the absence of any exposure to incompatible cells and are believed to arise from cross-sensitisation with bacterial antigens.

3 What is the rationale for administering anti-D antibodies to the mother?

Anti-D antibodies are administered to Rh D-negative women immediately after birth of a Rh D-positive child. Although the precise mechanism of action is not known it is believed that the antibodies coat the D-positive cells and mediate their removal before they can stimulate an antibody response. The effectiveness of the procedure is demonstrated by the dramatic fall in HDN deaths following the introduction of anti-D prophylaxis in the UK during 1967. Prior to this, some 850 deaths were attributed annually to HDN. Anti-D is now given to all Rh negative women following delivery, abortion (spontaneous or induced) and after any procedure that might produce a transplacental bleed, such as amniocentesis. Anti-D therapy has shifted the aetiology of HDN away from D-antigen sensitisation, with a higher proportion of present cases caused by anti-C, E, e and ABO antibodies.

4 Why is the incidence of ABO HDN much lower than the rate of maternofoetal ABO incompatiblity?

Some 20% of pregnancies are associated with a maternal–foetal ABO incompatibility, but the incidence of HDN is only a fraction of this number. Group A and group B mothers have anti-B and anti-A antibodies, respectively, but they are usually of the IgM class and therefore do not cross the placenta. The majority of ABO HDN occurs with group O mothers who have an increased incidence of IgG anti-B and anti-A antibodies. Most infants with ABO HDN are not profoundly anaemic and less than 0.05% require exchange transfusions.

■ CASE 24

Sixty-five-year-old Mr Brown presented to his GP in early January with cold extremities and malaise. He noted that his nose, ears, feet and hands became blue and numb in cold weather. Several weeks earlier he had developed a small area of ulceration over his left middle finger, which had since healed. On questioning he said the symptoms had been present for several years and always occurred during the winter months. Increasingly stiff and painful fingers and toes had prompted his visit to the doctor.

Recently he had noticed that his urine and faeces had been unusually dark, especially when the temperature was low. Mr Brown was not diabetic and had no history of claudication pain on exercise or at rest. On direct questioning he did not report any recent chest symptoms or any fever, weight loss, night sweats or alcohol related pain. There was no medical history of note and he was not taking any medication. He was a non-smoker and a moderate social drinker.

On examination Mr Brown was mildly jaundiced and had an area of acrocyanosis (purple discolouration) at the tip of his nose. His nail beds and sclera were pale. His hands and feet were pale and felt cold but peripheral pulses were present. There was no evidence of ulceration and sensation was normal. There was no oedema or lymphadenopathy. His liver and spleen were both palpable 1 cm below the costal margin but neither was tender. No other abdominal masses were present. His blood pressure was 145/85 and no heart murmurs could be heard. Respiratory examination was normal and he had no other signs of liver disease. The results of investigations are shown in *Figure 24.1*.

A diagnosis of primary (idiopathic) cold haemagglutinin disease (CHAD) was made as the history and investigations did not suggest a secondary cause.

QUESTIONS

1 What is the significance of the direct antiglobulin test (DAT)?
2 How can autoimmune haemolytic anaemia (AIHA) be classified?
3 What is the aetiology and pathogenesis of AIHA?
4 What treatment should be advised for CHAD?

Investigation	Result (normal range)
Haemoglobin (g/dl)	7.9 (13.5–18.0)
MCV (fl)	102 (78–96)
MCHC (%)	33 (30–34)
TIBC (mmol/l)	61 (45–72)
Serum iron (mmol/l)	25 (12–32)
Red cell folate (ng/l)	354 (160–640)
Serum B12 (ng/l)	750 (150–900)
White cell count (x 10⁹/l)	8.6 (4.0–11.0)
Platelet count (x 10⁹/l)	195 (150–400)
Blood film at +37°C	Mild ansiocytosis Mild reticulocytosis Mild spherocytosis No agglutination
Blood film at room temperature	Massive auto-agglutination
Direct antiglobulin test (DAT)	Weakly positive for C3 only on the red cell surface at 37°C. Increased agglutination at room temp
ESR	79 mm/hr
Total serum protein	71 g/l
Serum protein electrophoresis	Large γ-globulin peak

Serum immunoglobulins
  IgG (g/l)
  IgM (g/l)
	
	12.1 (5.4–16.1)
	5.8 (0.5–1.9)

Antibodies with specificity for the 'I' red cell antigen	Monoclonal kappa IgM found to react best at +4°C (titre 64 000)

Serum
  C3 (g/l)
  C4 (g/l)
	
	0.31 (0.75–1.65)
	0.39 (0.20–0.65)

Serum albumin (g/l)	41 (35–50)
Alkaline phosphatase (IU/l)	56 (30–300)
Aspartate transaminase (IU/l)	21 (5–35)
Serum bilirubin (μmol/l)	20 (3–17)
Haemoglobinuria	Positive
Chest X-ray	No abnormalities
Abdominal X-ray	No abnormalities

Fig. 24.1 Results of investigations.

■ **CASE 24** pp. 320–323

ANSWERS

1 What is the significance of the direct antiglobulin test?

The direct antiglobulin test (DAT) is used to detect antibody and/or complement which has become bound to the red cell surface *in vivo*. The antiglobulin reagent, which consists of a mixture of anti-immunoglobulin and anti-complement antibodies, is added to a sample of washed red cells from the patient. Agglutination of the cells is a positive result. Examples of conditions that are DAT positive include haemolytic disease of the newborn, autoimmune haemolytic anaemia and haemolytic transfusion reactions. Different antiglobulin agents with differing specificities (e.g. for IgG or IgM only) allow the test to determine the class of the immunoglobulin bound to the red cells. This technique can also be used to detect membrane bound complement.

The indirect antiglobulin test is used to detect the presence of unbound antibodies. Red cells are incubated with the patient's serum and are then washed with saline to remove excess antibodies. The antiglobulin reagent is then added and the sample observed for agglutination. The technique is most widely employed in the cross matching of blood where a prospective donor's red cells are incubated with the recipient's serum.

2 How can autoimmune haemolytic anaemia (AIHA) be classified?

Cold and warm variants of AIHA are compared and contrasted in *Figure 24.2*.

Feature	Warm AIHA	Cold AIHA	
		CHAD	Paroxysmal cold haemo-globinuria
Age of patient	Usually 35+	Usually 60+	Any age
Sex bias	F > M	F = M	F = M
Mechanism of red cell destruction	Extravascular haemolysis in liver + spleen	Extra- and intravascular haemolysis	Intravascular haemolysis
Class of antibody	IgG, usually IgG1 (rarely IgM, IgA)	IgM	IgG
Type of Ig response	Polyclonal	Monoclonal/ polyclonal	Polyclonal
Antibody specificity	Rh antigen (occasionally other, e.g. U, LW)	I antigen (i antigen in EBV infection)	P antigen
Antibody function *in vitro*	Incomplete agglutination	Complete agglutination	Biphasic haemolysis
Optimal reaction temperature	+37°C	0 → +4°C	0 → +4°C
Proteins on red cell surface	IgG 35% IgG + C3 55% C3 10%	C3 100%	C3 100%

Fig. 24.2 Classification of autoimmune haemolytic anaemia.

3 What is the aetiology and pathogenesis of AIHA?

Warm AIHA can be either idiopathic (55% of cases) or secondary in origin. Underlying causes include malignancies such as lymphoma and chronic lymphocytic leukaemia (18%), systemic lupus erythematosus (8%), infections (6%) and drugs such as methyldopa or mefenamic acid (5%). Idiopathic CHAD also accounts for 55% of cases. Secondary causes include *Mycoplasma* pneumonia (32%), lymphomas (10%) and infectious mononucleosis (3%). Idiopathic cases and those associated with malignancy involve monoclonal antibodies with the remainder being polyclonal. Fifty percent of paroxysmal cold haemoglobinuria (PCH) cases are idiopathic with the remaining 50% caused by measles, mumps or influenza virus infections.

Warm AIHA is characterised by the formation of IgG antibodies to the Rhesus system, usually the e antigen. Splenic macrophages bind the autoantibodies by Fc receptors and phagocytose the red blood cells. Those red cells with surface C3 can also be bound by macrophages via C3b receptors. A minority of cells are lysed in the intravascular compartment following activation of the full complement cascade and the formation of the membrane attack complex (MAC).

CHAD is characterised by the production of IgM antibodies to the I red cell antigen. These antibodies agglutinate the cells with increasing strength as the temperature is lowered, with optimal binding occurring at around +4°C. IgM bound to the red cells fixes complement in the peripheral circulation where the temperature is lower (especially in cold weather). When the cells circulate to a warmer area of the body, the antibodies dissociate leaving the C3 bound. Red cell destruction is then mediated by macrophages as in warm AIHA. Red cell agglutination in the periphery gives rise to Raynaud's phenomenom; peripheral arteriolar spasm causing pale and cold extremities. Secondary CHAD is most commonly associated with *Mycoplasma pneumoniae* infection where antibodies with typical anti-I activity is produced.

PCH is characterised by the production of Donath–Landsteiner IgG antibodies to the P red cell antigen. As in CHAD, the antibodies bind and fix complement at lower temperatures. However, when the cells are warmed to +37°C, they are lysed in the intravascular compartment by activation of the complement cascade.

4 What is the treatment for CHAD?

Primary treatment is to keep warm and this often improves symptoms. Thereafter alkylating agents such as chlorambucil may be helpful.

■ CASE 25

Twenty-four-year-old Miss Todd was seen by her GP with a 2-month history of relapsing and remitting tiredness and malaise. She had recently noticed a problem when speaking, which seemed to get worse with longer conversations. Reading had also become impossible because even short periods of focusing on a page induced blurring of her vision. Chewing food produced tiredness of her facial muscles and at times it even seemed an effort to keep her eyelids open. She usually attended regular fitness classes but her tolerance for exercise had dropped dramatically over the last month to the point that walking for more than 10 minutes drained her of all energy. She noted that her symptoms were worse around the time of her period, and that a recent cold had left her bed-bound for a week. She also reported a slight weight loss of 0.5 kg.

Miss Todd had no medical history of note with the exception of one normal pregnancy. There was no previous history of thyroid disease, pernicious anaemia or joint abnormalities. She had a 27-day menstrual cycle and did not report any menorrhagia. She worked as a secretary for a solicitor and had a happy home life with her partner and young son. Direct questioning did not reveal any evidence of depression and she did not have any headaches, black-outs, dysphagia, dizziness or alterations in sensation. A thorough systems review did not identify any other symptomatology.

On examination Miss Todd was within normal range for weight and height. She appeared slumped in her chair and had bilateral ptosis. There were no signs of anaemia or cervical lymphadenopathy. Her radial pulse was 72 beats/minute and her blood pressure was 115/75 mmHg. The remainder of her cardiovascular, respiratory and abdominal examinations were normal. Examination of her cranial nerves did not reveal any lesion but when she was asked to gaze upwards for some time, her ptosis became markedly worse. Sustained gaze in any direction for several minutes also produced diplopia, but no nystagmus. When asked to repeat a series of numbers for some minutes, her speech became increasingly dysarthric and palatal.

Further neurological examination did not reveal any muscle wasting, alterations in tone, or fasciculation. Power in all muscle groups was grade 4+ (range 0–5), but after repeated movement it decreased to grade 3 in the proximal muscle groups. All reflexes were present and she had flexor plantar responses. Her gait, coordination and sensory modalities were all normal. Administration of 2 mg of intravenous edrophonium produced no ill effects and a further dose of 10 mg was given. Within 2 minutes her proximal muscle power had improved to grade 4 in all groups. The results of investigations are shown in *Figure 25.1*.

A diagnosis of myasthenia gravis was made. An autoimmune screen for rheumatoid arthritis, systemic lupus erythematosus, pernicious anaemia and thyroiditis was performed because of the association of these disorders with myasthenia gravis. Miss Todd had anti-thyroid microsomal antibodies but her circulating T3 was normal and no action was therefore necessary. Chest imaging was used to detect the presence of any thymic abnormalities but none were identified.

Miss Todd was prescribed a course of pyridostigmine, an anticholinesterase agent, which produced an improvement for several months. Following a deterioration in her symptoms, azathioprine and corticosteroids were prescribed and she was referred for thymectomy. The procedure was performed without incident and remission was achieved.

QUESTIONS

1 How can myasthenia gravis be classified and what genetic associations exist?
2 What is the pathophysiology of myasthenia gravis?
3 How is the thymic pathology in myasthenia gravis related to the autoimmune process?

Investigation	Result (normal range)
Haemoglobin (g/dl)	12.6 (11.5–16.0)
Serum B12 (ng/l)	562 (150–900)
White cell count (x 10⁹/l)	12.6 (4.0–11.0)
Platelet count (x 10⁹/l)	259 (150–400)
Serum	
Sodium (mmol/l)	137 (134–145)
Potassium (mmol/l)	4.3 (3.5–5.0)
Chloride (mmol/l)	100 (95–105)
Calcium (ionised) (mmol/l)	1.19 (2.12–2.65)
Creatinine (µmol/l)	85 (70–150)
Urea (mmol/l)	3.9 (2.5–6.7)
Fasting blood glucose (mmol/l)	4.5 (4.0–6.7)
ESR	29 mm/hr
C reactive protein (mg/l)	7.5 (<5)
IgM rheumatoid factor	Negative
Anti-nuclear antibodies	Negative
Antibodies to extractable nuclear antigens	Negative
dsDNA binding activity	21%
Serum complement	
C3 (g/l)	0.98 (0.75–1.65)
C4 (g/l)	0.32 (0.20–0.65)
Serum T3 (nmol/l)	2.1 (1.2–3.0)
Anti-thyroglobulin antibodies	Negative
Anti-thyroid microsomal antibodies	Positive: titre 1 in 2500
Anti-parietal cell antibodies	Negative
Anti-intrinsic factor antibodies	Negative
Radioimmunoassay for anti-acetylcholine receptor antibodies	Positive
Repetitive nerve stimulation (prior to edrophonium) Decrease of >15% in amplitude of evoked muscle potential	
Pulmonary function test (prior to edrophonium) Decreased FVC and FEV1 for height and age, normal ratio	
AP and lateral chest X-ray and CT scan No mediastinal masses	

Fig. 25.1 Results of investigations.

■ **CASE 25**   pp. 327–328

ANSWERS

1 How can myasthenia gravis be classified and what genetic associations exist?

Myasthenia gravis (MG) can be divided into subgroups according to age, genetic associations, thymic pathology and clinical features (*Fig. 25.2*).

2 What is the pathophysiology of myasthenia gravis?

The underlying abnormality in myasthenia gravis, which was first demonstrated in the early 1970s, is a reduction in the number of acetylcholine receptors (AChRs) at the neuro-muscular junction. The postsynaptic membrane also shows a reduction in folding and the distance between the nerve end plate and the membrane is increased.

The nicotinic AChR is composed of five subunits (two α, one β, one δ and one γ or ε) which span the postsynaptic membrane. The subunits form a tube with a central cation channel which is closed in the resting state. The channel is opened when both ACh receptor sites on the α subunits are occupied, allowing the passage of cations. The receptors are in a continuous state of turnover with synthesis increasing if neuromuscular transmission is impaired.

Of patients with generalised MG, 90% have antibodies directed against the AChR, with the figure dropping to 60% in those with ocular disease only. Almost all are of the IgG class with all four subclasses present. AChR antibodies are hetero-geneous in their specificity within and between patients. Many, but not all, are directed against the main immunogenic region (MIR) of the α subunit with most of the remainder binding to other α epitopes. This heterogeneity explains the poor correla-tion between antibody titre and disease severity found in MG.

Three antibody mediated mechanisms are responsible for the diminution of AChRs: receptor blockade, cross-linking and complement-mediated damage. Up to 90% of patients with MG have antibodies which block the ACh binding sites on the AChR. A similar proportion of patients have antibodies capable of cross-linking AChRs. These receptor clusters are rapidly internalised by endocytosis and then degraded. IgG, C3 and the membrane attack complex (MAC) components of complement have been localised to the post-synaptic membrane. Furthermore, their deposition correlates with a low AChR concentration, confirming the relationship between complement activation and AChR loss.

3 How is the thymic pathology in myasthenia gravis related to the autoimmune process?

Some 15% of cases of myasthenia gravis are associated with a thymoma, an epithelial tumour which is locally invasive but rarely metastasises. A proportion of autoantibodies in MG cross-react with thymoma epithelial antigens. Furthermore, an epitope from the cytoplasmic domain of an AChR α sub-unit is expressed by these epithelial cells. It has been hypoth-esised that T lymphocytes become sensitised to AChR epitopes in the thymoma and circulate to the periphery to pro-mote the autoimmune response.

Thymectomy in patients with MG who do not have a thy-moma produces remission in 35% and improvement of symp-toms in a further 50%. The mechanism underlying these improvements is not known, although it has been suggested that removal of AChR epitopes putatively expressed in the myoid (muscle-like) cells of normal thymic tissue may reduce autosensitisation. The thymic medulla in such patients often contains T-cell areas surrounding secondary follicles with germinal centres indicative of local antibody production and thymic cell cultures can spontaneously synthesise AChR anti-bodies.

Subtype	Early onset	Late onset	Thymoma	Seronegative	Neonatal	D-penicillamine induced
% of cases	50%	20%	~15%	~15%	15% of offspring of myasthenic mothers	1% of rheumatoid cases treated with D-penicillamine
Age at onset (years)	<40	>40	Any	Any	At birth	Related to treatment
Sex ratio	F > M	M > F	M = F	M > F	M = F	Related to sex bias of RA
HLA associations	B8, DRw 3	B7, DR2	None	None	None	DR-1
Thymic pathology	Hyperplasia	Atrophy	Thymoma	Unknown	None	None
Pattern of weakness	Generalised	Generalised and ocular	Generalised	Generalised and ocular	Generalised	Generalised and ocular
Anti-AChR antibody titre	High	Low	Intermediate	None	Similar to mother	Low

Fig. 25.2 Subgroups of myasthenia gravis.

■ CASE 26

Mrs Rose was 52 when she noticed some red 'raw' areas around her umbilicus and also on her lips. She took no notice for a while but they became increasingly uncomfortable. She described the lesions as like being little blisters which then broke down to leave the red sore areas which then crusted over.

In the week before she was admitted to hospital, she developed widespread non-itchy red sore areas on her trunk and limbs. She also had lesions in her mouth and she generally felt ill with lethargy and loss of appetite. When she finally saw the doctor she had widespread erosions on her body, lips and scalp with haemorrhage and crusting. At that stage she was admitted to hospital.

A skin biopsy was performed and sent for analysis:

- Histopathology: 'Suprabasal acantholytic separation and vesiculation associated with eosinophil/neutrophil infiltrate. Separation of adjacent epidermal cells and a non-specific inflammatory infiltrate in the dermis. These findings are diagnostic of pemphigus.'
- Immunofluorescence: 'IgG and complement was seen within the epidermal tissue of the blister and at the margins. IgG was seen with the typical intercellular distribution.'

A diagnosis of pemphigus was made and further investigations carried out (*Fig. 26.1*). The patient was admitted to hospital and started on treatment with prednisolone 100 mg daily, intravenous fluids and erythromycin. After 48 hours of steroid treatment, considerable improvement was seen with no new lesions appearing and healing of the older lesions. The steroids were reduced gradually and the patient discharged from hospital on a maintenance dose. When the steroids were further reduced, new lesions appeared and azathioprine was added to the treatment regimen. On this, she remained well.

QUESTIONS

1 What is the immunological basis of damage in pemphigus?

2 Are the autoantibodies damaging, and, if so, what are the relevant autoantigens?

3 Which types of immunological diseases would you expect to be associated with pemphigus, and is there an HLA association?

4 How does immunosuppression affect treatment and prognosis of this disease, and can drug therapy be associated with the onset of pemphigus?

Investigation	Result (normal range)
Haemoglobin (g/l)	11.4 (11.5–16.0)
White cell count (x 10⁹/l)	6.0 (4.0–11.0)
Neutrophils (x 10⁹/l)	4.2
Lymphocytes (x 10⁹/l)	1.3
Eosinophils (x 10⁹/l)	0.72 (0.4–0.44)
Platelets (x 10⁹/l)	290 (150–400)
ESR	72 mm/hr
Serum IgE (IU/ml)	20 (3–150)
Serum	
Urea (mmol/l)	6.3 (2.5–6.7)
Sodium (mmol/l)	131 (134–145)
Potassium (mmol/l)	3.4 (3.5–5.0)
Chloride (mmol/l)	94 (95–105)
Skin swab	Group A streptococcus *Staphylococcus aureus*

Fig. 26.1 Results of investigations.

■ **CASE 26** pp. 326–327

ANSWERS

1 What is the immunological basis of damage in pemphigus?

Pemphigus vulgaris is a disease where intraepidermal, acantholytic vesicles and blisters develop on normal skin or mucosa. The separation of epidermal cells from one another is termed acantholysis. Pemphigus antibodies are directed against epidermal cells and can be detected in the serum and in affected skin. These antibodies disrupt the cohesive elements between these cells, the desmosomes. The condition is rare and there is no sex bias in those affected. There is a higher incidence in Jewish people.

The age of presentation is usually between 30 and 60 years but cases can occur in childhood or in old age. There is a strong HLA association of the disease. The aetiology is unknown but autoimmune disease and a slow virus infection have been suggested as possibilities. The differential diagnosis is from pemphigoid, dermatitis herpetiformis, epidermolysis bullosa acquisita and porphyria cutanea tarda.

2 Are the autoantibodies damaging, and, if so, what are the relevant autoantigens?

The histology of the pemphigus lesion shows acantholysis and deposition of IgG with an intercellular pattern. The predominant IgG subclass is IgG4 and the titre of these antibodies correlates directly with the severity of the disease. This suggests that there is a direct pathogenetic activity of the antibodies.

Animal studies show that when serum from patients with pemphigus is injected into neonatal mice, all the features of pemphigus are reproduced. Further experiments have shown that only IgG4 from patients will transfer the disease to mice and this subclass does not fix complement. Murine C3 is not detected in the lesions in mice after transfer of the disease.

The pemphigus vulgaris (PV) antigen has been isolated and is a 130 kDa polypeptide covalently bound to the 85 kDa peptide plakoglobin. This particular peptide is an integral constituent of desmosomes and tight junctions.

Antibodies raised against this antigen in rabbits also transfer the disease to mice, confirming the relevance of both the antibody and the antigen. In lesional but not normal skin, there is a deposition of complement. There is evidence of activation of the early components of the classical pathway but in addition, the later components – C5b-9 – the membrane attack complex (MAC), are seen. Complement does enhance epidermal cell detachment both *in vitro* and in animal passive transfer experiments.

The mechanism of activation of complement is unclear as the main autoantibody in pemphigus is IgG4, which is not complement fixing.

3 Which types of immunological diseases would you expect to be associated with pemphigus, and is there an HLA association?

The IgG autoantibodies in pemphigus give a characteristic staining of skin showing the typical intercellular distribution which is associated with the intra-epidermal blister. In this disease the antibody titre is proportional to the disease activity in the patient. Pemphigus is thus a true autoimmune disease, a fact that is reflected in its association with myasthenia gravis and thymoma and also systemic lupus erythematosus. It is also associated with pernicious anaemia and with Hodgkin's disease.

The HLA association of pemphigus is with HLA DR4/DQw3. However, there is also an association with DRw6/DQw1, which is strongly associated with the rare allele DQB1.3. This differs from the common DQβ-chain DQB1.1 by only a single amino acid. The significance of this lies in the relative risk of getting the disease by virtue of the frequency of various HLA types in the population.

The presence of DQB1.3 in Israelis gives an estimated relative risk of more than 100 compared to a relative risk of 2.6 for DRw6.

4 How does immunosuppression affect treatment and prognosis of this disease, and can drug therapy be associated with the onset of pemphigus?

Treatment of the disease is with high dose immunosuppressive therapy such as steroids, azathioprine, cyclophosphamide and cyclosporin. These therapies reduce the level of antibodies, promote healing and prevent the appearance of new lesions. Untreated pemphigus is fatal.

Once treated the course is unpredictable. Recurrent episodes of septicaemia may occur due to the immunosuppression. Unresponsive cases are sometimes helped by plasma exchange in conjunction with high dose corticosteroids.

Drugs are known to precipitate pemphigus. An autoimmune reaction to certain drugs such as captopril, isoniazid, indomethacin, propanolol and penicillamine can precipitate the production of antibodies to adhesive elements of keratinocytes within the epidermis and thus result in pemphigus.

For a comparison with bullous pemphigoid see *Figure 27.2* on page 54.

■ CASE 27

Sixty-five-year-old Mrs Read had complained for 2 weeks of an itchy rash on her arms, palms of her hands and soles of her feet and initially the rash was quite erythematous. Soon after this, she developed large tense blisters on her trunk and limbs. She also developed lesions on her vulva. With the eruption she sweated at night, had a fever and felt unwell. She had a past history of long standing plaque psoriasis which had not responded very well to topical treatment alone. She was therefore given intermittent courses of the retinoid, tigason (etretinate) by mouth. In 1994, the patient was given one of the newer retinoids, acitretin (neotigason) for 3 months. On this treatment she became nauseous and in fact her psoriasis became worse, and the new treatment was stopped. Some weeks before the blisters had erupted, she had been started again on the previous treatment, namely tigason.

When she was examined, she had large tense blisters on her limbs, trunk and vulva and was in considerable distress. There were no lesions in her mouth or on her scalp.

A biopsy taken from a lesion on her arm was sent for analysis
- Histopathology: 'Subepidermal bulla with an inflammatory infiltrate including eosinophils and necrotic keratinocytes. The features are those of bullous pemphigoid.'
- Immunofluorescence: 'Bright linear basement membrane zone fluorescence seen with C3 and to a lesser extent IgG. Typical of bullous pemphigoid.'

A diagnosis of bullous pemphigoid precipitated by tigason was made and further investigations performed (*Fig 27.1*). The patient was treated successfully with high dose corticosteroids in the form of oral prednisolone 60 mg daily for 2 weeks. The lesions improved with sloughing of the blisters, subsequent scab formation and scarring. The steroids were gradually reduced over the next few weeks to a maintenance dose sufficient to prevent new blisters from appearing.

QUESTIONS

1 What is the aetiology and pathology of bullous pemphigoid?
2 What is the type of immune response and where is the antibody directed?
3 What are the features of the skin lesion?
4 Does bullous pemphigoid occur in association with other diseases?
5 Are there any agents other than retinoids which can trigger bullous pemphigoid? What is the immune mechanism of this reaction in the skin?

Investigations	Results (normal range)
Haemoglobin (g/l)	13.3 (11.5–16.0)
White cell count (x 10⁹/l)	14.6 (4.0–11.0)
Eosinophils (x 10⁹/l)	4.38 (0.4–0.44)
Platelets (x 10⁹/l)	392 (150–400)
ESR	27 mm/hr
Serum IgE (IU/ml)	410 (3–150)
Creatinine (μmol/l)	96 (70–150)
Serum	
Urea (mmol/l)	6.2 (2.5–6.7)
Sodium (mmol/l)	139 (134–145)
Potassium (mmol/l)	4.1 (3.5–5.0)
Chloride (mmol/l)	98 (95–105)

Fig. 27.1 Results of investigations.

■ **CASE 27** pp. 326–327

ANSWERS

1 What is the aetiology and pathology of bullous pemphigoid?

This blistering disorder usually presents in elderly patients and has a chronic but relatively benign course where spontaneous healing may occur. Before corticosteroids became available, pemphigoid was fatal in one-third of subjects. Bullous pemphigoid is characterised by tense, sub-epidermal blisters on an erythematous base which arise spontaneously on the inner thighs, abdomen and flexures. Erosions may result with sub-epidermal separation. Mucosal blisters are rare. Early lesions prior to blistering are usually itchy and the erosions can be painful. There is often significant malaise with fever and generalised weakness.

Eosinophilia and a raised IgE are present in approximately half the patients. Histopathology of the skin shows a subepidermal blister with the roof consisting of the entire epidermis. The blister material consists of serum, fibrinous products and eosinophils. There may also be an inflammatory infiltrate in the surrounding dermis.

Electron microscopy shows antibody deposition at the dermo-epidermal junction between the cytoplasmic membrane of the basement cells and the lamina densa of the basement membrane.

2 What is the type of immune response and where is the antibody directed?

Direct immunofluorescence on skin biopsies from patients reveals linear and homogeneous deposits of immunoglobulins and complement components (C3) in the basement membrane beneath the epidermis. In 70% of cases, circulating antibodies to the basement membrane zone can be detected by indirect immunofluorescence using patients' serum on sections of normal skin. These pemphigoid antibodies are IgG and bind complement. Antibodies from patients with bullous pemphigoid bind to an antigen identified as a hemidesmosomal glycoprotein of 230 kDa.

However, the titre of antibody does not correlate with the severity of disease. The mechanism of bulla formation is thought to involve interaction between autoantibody, antigen, complement and leucocytes in a Type II hypersensitivity reaction.

3 What are the features of the skin lesion?

In the early lesions, lymphocytes are present and there is evidence of degranulated mast cells and eosinophils as well as a variety of chemotactic factors. Complement is deposited and membrane attack complexes (MAC) are present at the basement membrane zone. The presence of MAC demonstrates that complement activation proceeds to completion. The blister fluid confirms the relevance of complement activation in that it contains complement derived chemotactic factors and a reduced level of total haemolytic complement. Passive transfer of antibody to animals generally does not reproduce the disease. Thus, although there is some evidence for the damaging role of antibody in bullous pemphigoid, transfer experiments to support this hypothesis have not been positive.

4 Does bullous pemphigoid occur in association with other diseases?

The actual cause of pemphigoid is not clear but an autoimmune pathogenesis has been suggested because of the association of this condition with polymyositis, pemphigus vulgaris, dermatitis herpetiformis, systemic lupus erythematosus, ulcerative colitis, nephritis, polyarthritis, lichen planus and psoriasis. There is no evidence for an infective cause. Bullous pemphigoid can occur as a paraneoplastic phenomenon associated with malignancies of the prostate, lung or breast. In these situations, antibodies directed against the malignant cells may cross-react with the basement membrane zone of the skin.

5 Are there any agents other than retinoids which can trigger bullous pemphigoid?

Drugs such a salazosulphapyridine, penicillin, frusemide, diazepam and topical 5-fluorouracil have been implicated in the induction of bullous pemphigoid. Ultraviolet and X-rays have also precipitated this condition. A comparison of the major features of pemphigus and pemphigoid is shown in *Figure 27.2*.

Feature	Pemphigus	Pemphigoid
Age at onset	30–60	over 60
Bullous lesion	Intra-epidermal	Subepidermal
Characteristic autoantigen	Flaccid blisters intercellular substance (of epidermal pickle cells)	Tense bullae basement membrane (at dermo-epidermal junction)
Mouth involvement	>90%	<10%
HLA association	HLA DR4/DQw3 DRw6/DQw1 DQB1.3	None
Antibody titre	Proportional to disease activity	Not related to disease activity
IgE	Normal	Raised in 50%
Prognosis	Lethal if untreated	Lethal in 33% of untreated cases

Fig 27.2 A comparison of pemphigus vulgaris and bullous pemphigoid.

▊ CASE 28

Mr Franks, a 46-year-old farmer, eventually visited his doctor because over the past 18 months he had been feeling less well and also less able to do his work on the farm. In spite of eating well, he had lost some weight and developed a cough. He was a life long nonsmoker compared with his brother who worked on the farm with him and who smoked 40–60 cigarettes a day and had never had a cough. He was increasingly breathless and what worried him was that at spring time, he was coughing up some blood after he had put out the cattle. Like most farmers he had not had a really long holiday away from the farm for some years but had visited his family over Easter when he had felt much better. When he returned to the farm he had immediately come down with the 'flu'.

He had no previous history of chest problems affecting the lungs or heart. He had worked on the same farm for 10 years and considered himself to be physically fit. There was no family history of allergy (no hay fever, asthma or eczema), and none of his four children was atopic.

On examination, Mr Franks' chest expansion was reduced symmetrically and there were some fine end-inspiratory crackles at the lung bases. There was no finger clubbing and no lymph nodes were palpable. His cardiovascular system was normal. Simple lung function tests using a peak flow meter showed a peak expiratory flow rate of 380 l/min. A full blood count was normal and a Mantoux test negative. His doctor referred him to a chest specialist for further advice.

A chest X-ray was performed which showed bilateral reticulonodular shadowing in the middle and lower zones. Lung function tests showed a reduced forced expiratory volume in the first second (FEV1) and a reduced vital capacity (a restrictive defect), and the carbon monoxide gas transfer (diffusing capacity) was 60% reduced. A diagnosis of pulmonary fibrosis was made and further tests carried out to identify the cause (*Fig. 28.1*).

A diagnosis of extrinsic allergic alveolitis (EAA) was made. In this case, Mr Franks had inhaled thermophilic actinomycetes that were growing on his stored damp crops. This was especially prevalent in the spring when the hay was put out for the herd. This disease variant is therefore known as Farmer's Lung. Management consisted primarily of allergen avoidance using an industrial breathing mask. This patient needed oral corticosteroids to reduce the parenchymal inflammation in the lungs, and felt very much better.

QUESTIONS

1 Are precipitating antibodies characteristic of EAA?
2 What is the mechanism of lung damage?
3 Is pulmonary fibrosis likely to continue when the patient is removed from exposure to the antigen?
4 Does cigarette smoking have an effect on the course of the disease?

Investigation	Result *(normal range)*
Tests for precipitating antibodies 'precipitins'	Positive
Intradermal injection of *Micropolyspora faeni*	Arthus reaction
Bronchoalveolar lavage	Increased numbers of T lymphocytes and mast cells. CD8+ cells predominate with increased expression of MHC Class II antigens and activation markers
Lung biopsy	Granulomatous infiltrates of mononuclear cells, thickening of the alveolar walls with lymphocytic and plasma cell involvement
Immunofluorescent analysis of bronchial biopsy	Evidence for actinomycetes antigen in the alveolar spaces

Fig. 28.1 Results of investigations.

■ CASE 28   pp. 329–330

ANSWERS

1 Are precipitating antibodies characteristic of EAA?

Precipitating antibodies are considered to be the hallmark of EAA (hypersensitivity pneumonitis). This suggests that the mechanism of damage in EAA is a classical Type III hypersensitivity response due to the presence of local immune complexes following the inhalation of antigen. The evidence against a Type III mechanism is that precipitating antibody is found in approximately 50% of exposed but asymptomatic farmers. In experimental models of the disease in animals, transfer of serum from an affected to a normal animal does not transfer the disease when the recipient animal is exposed to the antigen. Interestingly, serum complement does not fall following bronchial challenge, suggesting that a Type III mechanism is not central to the disease. Lastly, vasculitis is not seen on biopsy of the lung as would be expected if immune complex deposition was the main immunopathological event. It appears that cellular immune responses constitute the main mechanism of injury.

For screening purposes it is still important to check for precipitating antibodies in a patient suspected of having EAA. If precipitins are present, then the crude dust extract contains the relevant antigen that the farmer is exposed to. Skin testing may demonstrate an immediate reaction, an Arthus reaction as well as a delayed response seen at 24–72 hours. As with the case of precipitins, this is not diagnostic as unaffected farmers with precipitins may show the same skin reactivity.

2 What is the mechanism of lung damage?

There are many biological effects of organic dusts. They are potent adjuvants and can stimulate alveolar macrophages directly. They can also activate the alternative pathway of complement which would provide a strong local reaction involving mediator production, increased permeability and increased chemotaxis of neutrophils and other cells into the lung parenchyma. They also contain toxic substances which can act locally.

Evidence for a cellular component in the damage can be shown in animal experiments. Animals immunised with the antigen can transfer sensitivity via cells to the recipient animal. Bronchial challenge of the recipient produces lesions in the lung similar to those seen in the human. Bronchoalveolar lavage (BAL) of sensitised animals shows lymphokine production as well as activated macrophages. Elevated levels of IL-1 can be found in extracts of lung granuloma, suggesting that macrophages and T cells within the lesions are active in cytokine production. IL-6 has also been shown at high levels in BAL fluid.

Studies involving the rabbit model of EAA have shown that the immunosuppressive drug cyclosporin A, when given before bronchial challenge, inhibits the appearance of the pathological lesions in the lungs. This is further evidence that cellular responses are critical in the lesions of hypersensitivity pneumonitis.

The ratio of CD4$^+$ to CD8$^+$ cells in BAL fluid of affected farmers shows a persistent reversal of ratios. In some subjects who have been studied following the cessation of their exposure to the antigen, the number of CD8$^+$ cells in the BAL has decreased, with the CD4$^+$ population increasing towards normal. The histopathology suggests a lymphocytic alveolitis.

3 Is pulmonary fibrosis likely to continue when the patient is removed from exposure to the antigen?

The classical presentation of EAA is of symptoms appearing some hours after exposure to antigen, e.g. mouldy hay. However, some farmers may present after several years with end stage fibrosis. They may have had some intercurrent 'fevers' associated with farming work, but have taken no notice of them. Current theories of fibrosing alveolitis are based on the idea that the damage to the endothelial or epithelial cells is associated with the accumulation of inflammatory cells in the interstitium of the lung and in the alveolar spaces. This leads to the release of mediators that stimulate collagen production by fibroblasts.

It is possible that the control of fibrous tissue deposition is associated with the epithelialisation of the bronchi and trachea. Where re-epithelialisation is prevented, such as by repeated local inflammation, fibrous tissue is laid down. Pulmonary epithelial cells are also involved in immunoregulation where they suppress clonal expansion of lymphocytes in the alveolar space. Thus, damage to epithelial cells may change the immunological environment, leading to a proliferation of lymphocytes which is a feature of both EAA and fibrosing alveolitis. Alveolar macrophages spontaneously release fibroblast mitogens when cultured *in vitro*, providing another potential stimulus to fibrosis.

4 Does cigarette smoking have an effect on the course of the disease?

There is no doubt that in Farmer's Lung and Bird Fancier's Lung, precipitating antibodies are more common in nonsmokers than smokers. The reason for this is not known but may reflect a generalised impairment of alveolar macrophage phagocytosis and antigen presentation in smokers. In a parallel series of observations it has been shown that cigarette smoking has a biphasic action on IgE levels. At a low level of smoking, IgE levels are enhanced but at high levels are suppressed. Occasionally, patients are seen who complain that they never suffered from allergic rhinitis when they smoked, only to have it appear when they stopped! This may reflect another effect on macrophage handling of antigen.

■ CASE 29

As a child, Yvonne had a number of sore throats for which the doctor had prescribed antibiotics, in particular penicillin. After a number of courses she developed a rash, was told that she had developed an allergy to penicillin and that she should not have it again. Fortunately, once she left school, she had very few further infections that needed antibiotic therapy.

Towards the end of a holiday abroad, at the age of 28, Yvonne developed acute cystitis with difficulty of micturition and some urinary frequency. When she got home she went to see her doctor, who gave her an antibiotic, trimethoprim, which she was to take for 8 days. She was, of course, not given penicillin.

She finished all the tablets and 3 days later developed a headache and some itchy lumps on her skin. The next day she had aching and swollen joints, mainly of the wrists and knees, although her hands were affected as well. She did not think that these symptoms had anything to do with the drug as she had already stopped taking it. She went to her doctor who confirmed that the rash was urticaria, but she also had a raised temperature and swollen glands in her neck. Examination of her urine showed evidence of protein.

The doctor asked for some further tests (*Fig. 29.1*) but in the meantime gave her some antihistamines with the warning that if these were not helpful she would need a course of corticosteroids. He diagnosed a drug allergy.

Her symptoms did not improve and she was started on oral prednisone. A renal biopsy was considered but not done because all the symptoms cleared following a course of corticosteroids.

Three weeks later Yvonne went for a check up and all her tests had returned to normal.

QUESTIONS

1 What is the likely mechanism of the reaction?
2 What non-immunological factors can lead to drug reactions?
3 Does a pre-existing drug allergy make the patient more likely to react to other drugs in the future?
4 What was the reason for asking for an autoantibody screen?

Investigation	Result (normal range)
Haemoglobin (g/dl)	14.1 (11.5–16.0)
White cell count (x 10^9/l)	10.1 (4.0–11.0)
Eosinophils (x 10^9/l)	1.45 (0.4–0.44)
Total lymphocytes (x 10^9/l)	2.2 (1.6–3.5)
ESR	34 mm/hr
C3 (g/l)	0.41 (0.75–1.65)
C4 (g/l)	0.09 (0.20–0.65)
ANA	Negative
Rheumatoid factor	Negative

Fig. 29.1 Results of investigations.

■ CASE 29   pp. 325–326

ANSWERS

1 What is the likely mechanism of the reaction?

The symptoms of rash, arthralgia and headache do have the hallmarks of an allergic drug response. However, the onset of the symptoms was after the drug had been discontinued, perhaps throwing doubt onto the causal relationship between drug intake and adverse response. Such a profile of symptoms is seen in the 'post-infection' syndrome and in that case is not caused by a drug reaction.

The delayed onset reflects the need for antigen to remain in the circulation for a prolonged period so that when sufficient antibody is synthesised, circulating antigen-antibody complexes are formed which 'precipitate' out into the various target tissues. Wherever the complexes are sited, complement can be fixed and local damage occur. This patient probably had damage to the glomeruli of the kidney as shown by the proteinuria as well as inflammation in the joints and skin. It is also possible that the urinary tract infection had not cleared and that was the origin of the proteinuria.

She also had abnormalities which showed that complement was being consumed – low C4 and C3 – as well as an increase in breakdown products, namely C3a. Named anaphylatoxins, C3a and C5a can directly release histamine from mast cells. This can lead to a confusing picture of a Type III hypersensitivity reaction presenting clinically as anaphylactic shock.

Old fashioned serum sickness reactions were seen with foreign protein injections such as anti-tetanus serum (ATS) which was made in horses. ATS was given when there was a danger of tetanus to provide passive immunity to the patient whilst active immunisation was being given. Blood products can also give a serum sickness syndrome.

2 What non-immunological factors can lead to drug reactions?

A variety of drugs can cause reactions by activating effector pathways by non-immunological means. Some drugs, such as opiates, can cause the release of mediators from mast cells by direct action on the cell, without the involvement of IgE. Some compounds, such as X-ray contrast material given intravenously in order to visualise the excretion pattern of the kidney, activate the alternative pathway of complement and thereby produce anaphylatoxins, C3a and C5a. As mentioned above, this can lead to anaphylactic shock. Other drugs such as aspirin and non-steroidal anti-inflammatory drugs (NSAIDs) alter arachidonic acid pathways and can again produce anaphylactic shock. There is a well described triad of asthma, nasal polyps and aspirin sensitivity. These patients are at risk of acute status asthmaticus if they take an aspirin or other NSAID.

Other reactions can be produced by overdose where the symptoms are predictable and due to the main action of the drug. This may not be deliberate but due to the poor excretion of the drug by the patient or its slow breakdown. Secondary effects are often seen and these represent actions of the drugs that are not the ones for which the drug is given. Examples of this are the alopecia, gut problems and bone marrow toxicity of many immunosuppressive compounds.

Other factors relate to the 'ecology' of the patient taking the drugs. Broad spectrum antibiotics change the bacterial flora in the gut and often lead to an overgrowth of candida in the mouth, gastrointestinal tract or vagina. Drug interactions can also lead to clinical problems. Probenecid given for gout interferes with penicillin excretion by the kidney. Phenytoin given for epilepsy interferes with folate metabolism. It has also been reported to lead to reduced levels of IgA if given long term.

Some drugs actually make the pre-existing disease worse. This is best seen in skin disease where lithium given for manic-depressive illnesses can exacerbate both acne and psoriasis.

3 Does a pre-existing drug allergy make the patient more likely to react to other drugs in the future?

If a patient has already had an allergic reaction to penicillin, they are 10 times more likely to react to other antibiotics. The reverse is also true in that if a patient has already reacted to other antimicrobials, he or she is more likely to react to penicillin. There are definable risk factors for drug allergy such as genetic background, metabolic status, concurrent drug therapy and the role of the illness itself, such as HIV infection or autoimmune disease, in altering the handling of drugs. This can be seen in patients taking aminophylline for asthma who have a virus infection. The virus reduces the degradation of aminophylline by the cytochrome P450 enzyme system, increases the half life and can cause toxicity.

4 What was the reason for asking for an autoantibody screen?

The patient presented with a rash, painful joints and evidence of renal damage as shown by proteinuria. A possible diagnosis was systemic lupus erythematosus (SLE). In this instance it could have been induced by drugs when the antinuclear antibody would have been positive. A number of drugs, especially hydralazine and procainamide, are capable of inducing antinuclear antibodies in a significant proportion of patients taking them – in the region of 60%. In most of the patients the antibodies are harmless and may remain at a high titre even when the drugs have been discontinued for years.

In a small percentage of patients, a clinical syndrome resembling SLE does develop. The main symptoms in these instances are pulmonary and polyserositis but there is a general lack of kidney or nervous system involvement. It would be unlikely on clinical grounds that Yvonne had drug induced SLE and her antinuclear antibodies were negative. The mechanisms by which these drugs induce the autoantibodies is unknown. The lupus inducing drugs can be given to patients with pre-existing SLE without making the condition worse.

■ CASE 30

Mr Jackson, a 31-year-old Irishman, presented to his GP with a 3-month history of malaise, anorexia, weight loss, mild diffuse abdominal pain and diarrhoea. Over the last fortnight he had vomited every other day and had developed an itchy, blistering rash on the extensor surfaces of his knees and elbows. He had not vomited any blood or had any obvious bleeding from the gut. Recently, mealtimes were accompanied by bloating and he noted his stools were also paler than normal. He was not taking any medication and had not travelled abroad. His relatives lived in Ireland and he was unable to recall any family history of disease. He did not complain of muscle cramps, paraesthesia or bruising.

On examination, Mr Jackson was underweight for his height and had finger clubbing, several aphthous mouth ulcers, and angular cheilitis. He had a vesicular rash on the extensor surfaces of his elbows and knees. There was no jaundice or oedema, but he was clinically anaemic. He had a mildly distended and non-tender abdomen and normal bowel sounds. No masses were felt on palpation or on rectal examination, and there was no evidence of per rectum bleeding. Mr Jackson's doctor decided to refer him to a gastroenterologist for further evaluation. The results of investigations are shown in *Figure 30.1*.

Mr Jackson had combined iron and folate deficiency anaemia and low serum albumin. His mild hypocalcaemia was compensated by a degree of secondary hyperparathyroidism. The gastroenterologist identified his rash as dermatitis herpetiformis, and this, combined with the history and laboratory evidence of malabsorption, led to a provisional diagnosis of coeliac disease (gluten enteropathy).

A jejunal biopsy was performed and the sample sent for histological examination. The presence of subtotal villous atrophy, elongated crypts and a dense inflammatory infiltrate was strongly suggestive of coeliac disease. The diagnosis was further confirmed by positive enzyme-linked immunosorbent assays (ELISAs) for serum IgA antibodies to endomysium, gliadin and reticulin.

Mr Jackson was referred to a dietician who outlined a gluten-free diet and provided calcium, folate and iron supplements. In the next 3 months he gained several kg in weight and his other symptoms improved considerably. At a follow-up appointment his endomysium, gliadin and reticulin antibody levels were lower than those at presentation and a repeat biopsy showed an improvement in jejunal architecture. Other indices, including his serum albumin, calcium, haemoglobin and clotting, were within normal limits. Mr Jackson was advised to observe a gluten-free diet for life and regular follow-up appointments were arranged because of the increased risk of small bowel malignancy in patients with coeliac disease.

QUESTIONS

1 What is the aetiology of coeliac disease?
2 What is the immunopathology of coeliac disease?
3 Is the patient's antibody status sufficient to make the diagnosis of coeliac disease?
4 Can other foods cause the same clinical picture?

Investigation	Result (normal range)
Haemoglobin (g/dl)	10.1 (13.5–18.0)
MCV (fl)	82 (78–96)
MCH (pg)	25 (27–32)
TIBC (mmol/l)	60 (45–72)
TIBC saturation	<10%
Serum iron	7 mmol/l
Red cell folate (ng/l)	135 (160–640)
Serum B12 (ng/l)	426 (150–900)
Blood film	Microcytes Oval macrocytes Howell–Jolly bodies
Platelet count (x 10⁹/l)	280 (150–400)
White cell count (x 10⁹/l)	15.2 (4.0–11.0)
Neutrophils (x 10⁹/l)	8.4 (2.0–7.5)
Eosinophils (x 10⁹/l)	0.46 (0.4–0.44)
Total lymphocytes (x 10⁹/l)	9.9 (1.6–3.5)
Serum immunoglobulins	
IgG (g/l)	18.2 (5.4–16.1)
IgM (g/l)	0.4 (0.5–1.9)
IgA (g/l)	3.9 (0.8–2.8)
IgE (IU/ml)	51 (3–150)
Serum	
Sodium (mmol/l)	134 (134–145)
Potassium (mmol/l)	3.4 (3.5–5.0)
Calcium (ionised) (mmol/l)	1.65 (2.12–2.65)
Phosphate (mmol/l)	1.26 (0.8–1.45)
Chloride (mmol/l)	95 (95–105)
Serum parathyroid hormone	0.89 (µg/l)
Liver function tests:	
Serum albumin (g/l)	29 (35–50)
Alkaline phosphatase (IU/l)	64 (30–300)
Aspartate transaminase (IU/ml)	37 (5–35)
Serum bilirubin (µmol/l)	12 (3–17)
Prothrombin time (secs)	19 (10–14)
Activated partial thromboplastin time (secs)	55 (35–45)
ESR	10 mm/hr
Faecal fat (g/24hr)	27 (<6g/24hr)
Faecal blood	Trace
Stool culture	Negative
Abdominal X-ray	Small bowel distension

Fig. 30.1 Results of investigations.

■ **CASE 30**   p. 329

ANSWERS

1 What is the aetiology of coeliac disease?

Coeliac disease (CD) is a disorder of the small intestine characterised by villous atrophy and malabsorption caused by an adverse reaction to dietary gluten (a water insoluble component of flour). The UK prevalence is 1 in 2000 but in some areas, e.g. the West of Ireland, it is as high as 1 in 300. The disease can occur at any age but two peaks are found between the ages of 1–5 and 20–40.

Recent studies identified the toxic moiety as the α-gliadin component of gluten. Challenging coeliac patients with polypeptides from α-gliadin suggests that toxicity may be restricted to amino acids 31–49. Sequencing data have also demonstrated that α-gliadin shares a 12 amino acid sequence with the non-structural E1B peptide of human adenovirus 12. Challenges with a sequence containing this peptide (amino acids 202–220) produce only minor histological changes in a minority of patients. The role of molecular mimicry in CD therefore remains unclear.

The prevalence of CD amongst first-degree relatives of sufferers is 10–15%. Susceptibility is conferred, at least in part, by the HLA-D region of the MHC II genes. Eighty percent of affected individuals have the haplotype HLA-B8, DR3, DQw2. In Italy and Spain, the haplotype is HLA-DR7, DQw2. However, the finding that the disease concordance rate for identical twins is 75% but that it is only 40% for HLA identical siblings suggests a role for another gene outside the HLA locus.

CD is associated with other immunological disorders. Isolated IgA deficiency (Case 7), which shares a common genetic linkage, has an increased prevalence of 1 in 50 subjects. Ninety-five percent of patients with dermatitis herpetiformis (DH) have an abnormal jejunal mucosa, most commonly patchy subtotal villus atrophy. This vesicular rash, characterised by subepidermal deposits of IgA and C3, usually responds to a gluten-free diet. The specificity of the IgA in the skin is unknown. The majority of patients also have the HLA-B8, DR3, DQw2 haplotype.

High molecular weight glutenin (HMW-g), a component of gluten, has been shown to have structural similarities to human elastin. IgA antibodies which cross-react with HMW-g and elastin have been identified in the sera of patients with CD and DH. This has led to the hypothesis that DH may be an autoimmune disease caused by cross-reactivity between dietary glutenin and dermal elastin.

Extrinsic allergic alveolitis, insulin dependent diabetes mellitus, Addison's disease, systemic lupus erythematosus, rheumatoid arthritis, Sjögren's syndrome and autoimmune thyroid disease also have an increased prevalence in CD. In addition, CD can be considered a pre-malignant condition because of the increased risk of malignant T-cell lymphoma and carcinoma of the jejunum, oesophagus and pharynx.

2 What is the immunopathology of coeliac disease?

The mucosal lesion is characterised by depletion of the enterocyte brush border population with increased replication of crypt epithelial cells. The latter leads to crypt hyperplasia and elongation. The loss of mucosal architecture is responsible for the subsequent malabsorption seen in these patients. These changes are initiated by an inflammatory cell infiltrate of T and B lymphocytes, plasma cells and macrophages. The epithelium is infiltrated with $CD8^+$, $CD3^+$ α/β and $CD8^-$, $CD3^+$ γ/δ ICAM-1/LFA-1 negative T lymphocytes. $CD4^+$, $CD3^+$, LFA-1/ICAM-1$^+$ positive T cells are restricted, with occasional macrophages, to the lamina propria. Gliadin-specific $CD4^+$ cells are found in the mucosa and most are restricted to the HLA-DQ dimer.

Genetic linkage to the HLA loci, the nature of the mucosal infiltrate and an association with other immunological disorders point to an immune pathogenesis for CD. The role of intestinal and serum antibodies to toxic components of gluten is equivocal as they are also found in a proportion of normal controls. Both immune complex and cell mediated mechanisms have been proposed but, as yet, the origin of the mucosal damage remains unclear.

3 Is the patient's antibody status sufficient to make the diagnosis of coeliac disease?

Three antibody specificities can aid the diagnosis of CD. IgG and IgA antibodies to gliadin have a high specificity but poor sensitivity. Anti-reticulin IgA antibodies have an almost 100% specificity but intermediate sensitivity. IgA antibodies to endomysium (IgA-EMA), the loose connective tissue found surrounding muscle fibres, are the most reliable serological marker for the diagnosis of coeliac disease. IgA-EMA titres also reflect variations in dietary gluten and correlate well with intestinal pathology. Current practice in the UK is to use a combination of jejunal biopsy and antibody status to confirm the diagnosis.

4 Can other foods cause the same clinical picture?

Other foods have been implicated in gastrointestinal villous atrophy: for example, eggs, milk and chicken. It is thought that with these foods the disease is not so long-lasting or severe.

CASE 32

Twenty-five-year-old Miss Noakes had a very busy job with a large industrial firm and also looked after the home of her parents who were both invalids. She was very house proud and kept the house extremely clean. Over some weeks she had developed a rash on various parts of her body, but particularly on the hands and wrist, around the neck and on both ear lobes. The rash slowly became worse and she consulted a dermatologist.

As a child she had suffered from atopic eczema and in her teens had facial acne for which she was given tetracycline; there was no other medical history of note. On examination, the rash consisted of erythema and small blisters. There was marked excoriation because of the itching. Her hands were red, scaly and dry and the rash there looked quite different to the areas on her neck and ears. The dermatologist suspected a contact hypersensitivity, so applied a battery of standard contact sensitisers as patch tests to her back and examined the sites after 2 and 4 days. The standard battery included rubber, cosmetics, plant extracts, perfumes, metals, make-up and so on. The strongly positive reactions were to rubber and nickel.

Miss Noakes was advised to stop wearing rubber gloves when washing up and cleaning, and substitute ones with a cotton lining. When questioned more closely concerning her jewellery, she mentioned that she had recently been given a set of ear-rings, necklace and watch by her current boyfriend and these were presumed to be the cause of her contact dermatitis. She was prescribed a mild corticosteroid cream and advised to stop wearing that jewellery. She had no further episodes of skin allergy since that time. It was suggested that she should wear only expensive jewellery in future!

QUESTIONS

1 What are the characteristics of the antigen in the jewellery?
2 What is the evidence that Type IV hypersensitivity is involved in contact eczema?
3 What is the mechanism of elicitation of contact eczema?
4 What is the mechanism for down regulating the response to contact allergens?

■ **CASE 32** pp. 341–342

ANSWERS

1 What are the characteristics of the antigen in the jewellery?

The reaction of contact allergy is a classical example of Type IV hypersensitivity. The reaction itself is one of eczema where the external agent comes into contact with the skin. The most common causative agents are haptens such as metals, chromate and nickel, as well as chemicals, poison ivy and poison oak. Drugs that are topically applied can also lead to contact reactions.

Haptens are small molecules that are too small themselves to elicit an immunological response. They often have a molecular weight in the region of 1 kDa. When these small molecules penetrate the epidermis they form covalent bonds with body proteins and produce the immunogenic hapten-carrier complex. Only a small proportion of people who come into contact with nickel become sensitised and it is difficult to predict the sensitising capacity of the hapten from its chemical structure.

There is some correlation with the number of haptens attached to the carrier, the ability of the molecule to penetrate the skin and whether the contact agent has unsaturated carbon bonds that can be oxidised to provide links for further bonding. Some contact agents such as dinitrochlorobenzene (DNCB) have the ability to sensitise virtually all people and can therefore be used as a measure of cell mediated immunity in patients suspected of immune deficiency. Almost all the applied DNCB becomes attached to epidermal cells through the -NH_2 group of the amino acid lysine. The recognition of the hapten-carrier by the T cell is specific for the conjugate itself and does not involve separate recognition of the hapten and carrier as occurs in antibody formation.

2 What is the evidence that Type IV hypersensitivity is involved in contact eczema?

Extensive research has been carried out into the pathology of contact eczema and there are a number of clear lines of evidence that cell mediated reactions are crucially involved in the lesions in the skin.

- Lymphatics are necessary for the induction of the contact eczema lesions in the skin. If a skin flap has the lymphatics cut, then sensitisation following epicutaneous agents does not occur.
- As with other cell mediated reactions, sensitivity can be transferred from an immunised animal to a normal one by cells and not by serum.
- Elicitation of contact hypersensitivity needs a vascular supply to the challenged area. A contact eczema will result in the skin site only if the animal has been sensitised at a distant area.
- If biopsies are taken of an area of skin following the application of a sensitising chemical, there is an increase in the veiled cells in the draining lymph node and a substantial increase in the Langerhans' cells in the paracortical area of the draining lymph nodes.

- When lymphocyte activation is performed *in vitro*, epidermal Langerhans' cells can act as antigen presenting cells for the T lymphocytes of allergic subjects.

It is interesting that if the area of skin to be sensitised is pre-treated with ultraviolet irradiation, sensitisation does not occur and the number of Langerhans' cells is very much reduced. In addition, when these cells are placed in culture, they no longer act as APCs thus explaining the action of UVB. These several lines of evidence show that it is the cellular response that induces the lesions of contact eczema.

3 What is the mechanism of elicitation of contact eczema?

There are two main phases of the contact hypersensitivity reaction. The first is sensitisation which can take up to 2 weeks. During this stage the hapten has combined with the carrier protein and been processed by the Langerhans' cells which are in the epidermis. These then migrate to the paracortical area of the draining lymph node where MHC class II molecules present the antigen to CD4$^+$ lymphocytes leading to clonal expansion.

The second, the elicitation phase, also involves the Langerhans' cells. Following the application of the contact agent to the skin, there is a fall in the resident population of Langerhans' cells in the epidermis. Presentation of the antigen occurs in the skin and local lymph node with the release of cytokines from many types of cells. There is also evidence of mast cell degranulation after contact with the allergen and this leads not only to mediator release but to further production of cytokines as well. TNFα and IL-1 induce adhesion molecules on endothelial cells which produce a signal for mononuclear cell migration into the skin.

One of the early cellular changes is the finding of mononuclear cells in the epidermis, the peak of cell infiltration being reached at 48–72 hours. The lymphocytes that are present are CD4$^+$ with a small number of CD8$^+$. Because of the amplification of cell infiltration by cytokines, the cell recruitment is not antigen specific.

4 What is the mechanism for down regulating the response to contact allergens?

The clinical reaction to the application of a contact allergen will begin to fade after 2 days and will clear after a week. This is the result of many actions in the skin. After some days the hapten-carrier complex will be degraded and the antigen drive will be reduced. Prostaglandins of the E type are produced by keratinocytes and macrophages in the skin and these in turn will down regulate both IL-1 and IL-2. TGFβ also down regulates the stimulatory effects of IL-1 and IL-2. Cytokines also inhibit the migration of macrophages from the test site to help prevent the spread of the allergic response. The expression of class II molecules, which will also be affected by IL-10, in turn amplifies the suppression of cytokine production and will further inhibit the proliferation of TH1 cells.

■ CASE 33

Three-year-old Kanti was seen by his GP with a 3-month history of malaise, reduced appetite and a weight loss of 2 kg. Over the past month he had experienced episodes of fever and sweating at night and had developed a productive cough. He did not have any chest pain, dyspnoea, wheezing or haemoptysis. The medical history of note included otitis media which had responded to antibiotic therapy. He had no previous history of prolonged respiratory tract infections or asthma. His mother was well but his father had a history of 'chest trouble'. Further inquiry did not reveal any additional symptoms and his mother was unaware of him receiving any immunisations.

On examination, Kanti was underweight for his height and age, and he coughed during the consultation. He was clinically anaemic but had no jaundice, clubbing or lymphadenopathy. His temperature was 37.4 °C, his radial pulse 110 beats/min and his blood pressure 95/55 mmHg. No evidence of a BCG vaccination site could be found. A respiratory examination revealed an area of dull percussion note, reduced air entry and wheezes over the right upper zone. The remainder of his cardiovascular examination was normal. Examination of his abdomen did not reveal any tenderness or palpable masses. His spine was similarly free of masses and was not tender to percussion. The results of investigations are shown in *Figure 33.2*.

A clear diagnosis of pulmonary tuberculosis was made. The organism was sent to the reference laboratory for sensitivities; which reported no evidence of drug resistance. Kanti was started on a course of isoniazid and rifampicin (both bactericidal agents) for 9 months, with ethambutol (a bacteriostatic agent) and pyrazinamide (bactericidal) for the first 2 months. Pyridoxine (vitamin B6) was also prescribed throughout. Side effects of this regimen include hepatic dysfunction and so regular liver function tests were performed. His family were also advised to attend for screening. Kanti's symptoms improved and a subsequent chest X-ray taken at 12 months showed some fibrosis of the right middle lobe with volume loss of the right lung, but no evidence of active disease.

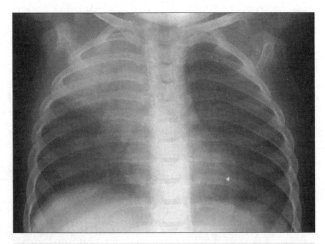

Fig. 33.1 Chest X-ray showing right upper lobe consolidation and an enlarged right hilum.

QUESTIONS

1 What is the epidemiology of tuberculosis infection?
2 What is the immunopathology of tuberculosis?
3 What clinical outcomes are possible following a primary infection?

Investigation	Result *(normal range)*
Haemoglobin *(g/dl)*	11.2 *(13.5–18.0)*
MCV *(fl)*	82 *(78–96)*
MCH *(pg)*	30 *(27–32)*
TIBC *(mmol/l)*	60 *(45–77)*
Serum iron *(mmol/l)*	21 *(12–32)*
Red cell folate *(ng/l)*	410 *(160–640)*
Serum B12 *(ng/l)*	320 *(150–900)*
Blood film	Normocytic red cells
Platelet count *(x 10⁹/l)*	320 *(150–400)*
White cell count *(x 10⁹/l)*	16.1 *(6.8–10.0)*
Serum	
Sodium *(mmol/l)*	139 *(134–145)*
Potassium *(mmol/l)*	4.3 *(3.5–5.0)*
Chloride *(mmol/l)*	98 *(95–105)*
Creatinine *(μmol/l)*	110 *(70–150)*
Urea *(mmol/l)*	2.9 *(2.5–6.7)*
Liver function tests	
Serum albumin *(g/l)*	45 *(35–50)*
Alkaline phosphatase *(IU/l)*	201 *(30–300)*
Aspartate transaminase *(IU/ml)*	31 *(5–35)*
Serum bilirubin *(μmol/l)*	7 *(3–17)*
Random blood glucose *(mmol/l)*	7.2 *(<10.0)*
ESR	21 mm/hr
Chest X-ray *(Fig. 33.1)*	Right hilar enlargement. Area of consolidation in the right upper zone
Blood cultures	Negative
Ziehl–Neelsen stain of sputum smear	*M. tuberculosis* bacilli
Sputum culture	Positive for *M. tuberculosis* at 6 weeks
Intradermal injection of purified protein derivative of *M. tuberculosis*	Strongly positive Mantoux test, 10 mm induration, 10 mm of erythema

Fig. 33.2 Results of investigations.

■ CASE 33   pp. 345–346, 135

ANSWERS

1 What is the epidemiology of tuberculosis infection?

The WHO estimates that some 50–100 million people a year become infected with *Mycobacterium tuberculosis*. At any one time there are probably 20 million active cases worldwide. Tuberculosis (TB) has the highest morbidity and mortality of any infection, with approximately 3 million deaths annually. The prevalence of TB declined steadily in the Western world throughout the latter half of this century but in the mid-1980s this trend was reversed. The number of new cases in the USA increased by 18% between 1985–91.

This resurgence has paralleled the world-wide increase in HIV infection. The incidence of TB is 500 times higher in HIV-positive individuals than in the general population. This however is not the only reason for the increase. The tubercle bacillus is almost exclusively transmitted by air. Water droplets from the lung released during coughing or normal breathing contain the organism. Thus, crowded urban living conditions and low socioeconomic status are positively associated with an increased incidence of TB. Other risk factors include age (the young and the old), immunodeficiency (e.g. HIV infection, corticosteroid therapy), previous lung disease (e.g. silicosis) and any chronic debilitating illness.

2 What is the immunopathology of tuberculosis?

Following inhalation, tubercle bacilli are internalised by alveolar macrophages (AM), which are usually in an activated state due to nonspecific stimulation from inhaled particles. At this stage many organisms are destroyed by the production of oxygen and nitrogen radicals and the addition of lysosomal enzymes to the phagosome. *M. tuberculosis* has the capacity to inhibit lysosomal fusion, hence a proportion survive and divide. The macrophage then ruptures, releasing the bacilli, which are ingested by further AM and blood derived monocytes. The latter, which become the predominant source of phagocytes in the lesion, are in an inactivated state. The bacilli are therefore able to survive within the cells, where they multiply logarithmically.

T cells recruited into the lesion by the chemoattractant IL-8 activate the immature macrophages by producing IL-2 and IFNγ. The macrophages mature into epithelioid cells and some fuse to form Langerhans' giant cells. This cellular mass undergoes caseating necrosis, a process largely orchestrated by cytotoxic T cells. Macrophage free radical and TNFα production is also of importance. The pivotal role of cytotoxic T lymphocytes in the immune response to TB is confirmed by the finding that mice depleted of CD8⁺ T cells die rapidly of mycobacterial infection.

The onset of necrosis corresponds to the acquisition of a delayed hypersensitivity reaction. If the patient is given an intradermal injection of mycobacterial proteins at this stage, the Koch phenomenon is observed. Twelve hours after the injection, CD4⁺ and CD8⁺ T cells migrate to the area, followed at 48 hours by macrophages. Bacterial antigens are presented by macrophages to T cells previously sensitised to bacilli in the lung. The area of skin indurates and heals rapidly.

This reaction is the basis of the Mantoux test which determines previous exposure to the bacillus or the BCG vaccine.

Following caseation, activated macrophages in an immunocompetent host are able to ingest and destroy bacilli at the periphery of the necrotic tissue. The lesion becomes 'walled off' and eventually undergoes fibrosis. Those with weaker cell mediated immunity are unable to activate these peripheral macrophages and hence the lesion enlarges. Bacilli lodged in hilar lymph nodes drain into the venous system and are able to disseminate throughout the body.

In a proportion of patients, regardless of immunocompetence, the caseated lesion undergoes liquefaction. This medium is ideal for bacterial replication, and the bacilli multiply in the extracellular environment. The availability of large quantities of antigen leads to necrosis of the bronchi by a cell mediated response. Cavities form and the bacillus is able to reinfect other areas of the lung via the airways.

3 What clinical outcomes are possible following a primary infection?

See *Figure 33.3*.

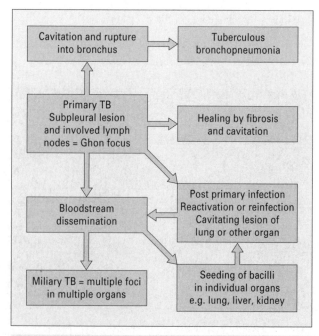

Fig. 33.3 Possible outcomes of a primary infection with *M. tuberculosis*.

CASE 34

As a child, Mr James lived in the family compound and went to school in the local village. He was said to have had some skin lesions when young – a macule on his chest wall about 5 cm in diameter. This disappeared after 6 months. As an adult he emigrated to the southern states of the USA.

He first noticed loss of his eyebrows and then thickening of his nostrils, ears and cheeks. There were many vague-edged, hypopigmented maculae on his chest and arms and his skin seemed to become thicker. Over several months he had noticed areas of anaesthesia on his hands and although his muscle power was normal, cuts and other lesions developed on his hands, although he did not notice them until later. The cuts on his fingers were infected and there was some damage to the bones in his hands.

His family began to see a change in the shape of his face which became 'leonine'. He had a continual nasal discharge and was sent to an otorhinolayrngologist and dermatologist for diagnosis.

On examination he did indeed have a leonine look to his face and there were multiple lesions on his hands, with some absorption of the terminal phalanges. There was also infiltration of the skin, with one annular lesion on his chest wall. Some of the nerves felt obviously thickened. His hands and feet showed patchy anaesthesia. The initial results are given in *Figure 34.1*. A diagnosis of leprosy was made and Mr Jones was treated with dapsone, rifampicin and clofazimine.

After some months of treatment he felt ill and developed red lesions scattered all over his body, which were tender to touch and raised above the surrounding skin surface. He also had painful joints at the same time. He was given further treatment for this reaction which was diagnosed as erythema nodosum leprosum.

QUESTIONS

1 What is the classification of leprosy?
2 Why has the patient developed erythema nodosum leprosum (ENL)?
3 What is the treatment for ENL?
4 Are there any genetic associations with the clinical response to *Mycobacterium leprae*?

Investigation	Result *(normal range)*
Haemoglobin *(g/dl)*	15.9 *(13.5–18.0)*
White cell count *(x 10⁹/l)*	8.9 *(4.0–11.0)*
X-ray of hands	Cyst in proximal metacarpal of left index finger
X-ray of chest	Normal
Nasal mucus smear	Multiple acid-fast bacilli present
Skin biopsy	The dermis was heavily infiltrated with foamy histiocytes laden with leprosy bacilli. The epidermis contained very few bacilli and there was no obvious presence of lymphocytes

Fig. 34.1 Results of investigations.

■ **CASE 34** pp. 348–351, 329, 135

ANSWERS

1 What is the classification of leprosy?

Humans respond in a variety of ways to infection with *Mycobacterium leprae*. The combination of the immunological response and host characteristics will determine the type of disease that is seen. There are two polar groups of patients in leprosy: full tuberculoid (TT) and full lepromatous (LL). Between these two types there is borderline (BB); intermediate between BB and the polar groups are borderline tuberculoid (BT) and borderline lepromatous (BL).

The two extreme forms of leprosy, TT and LL, are characterised by the presence or absence of cell mediated immunity (CMI) and antibody.

At the TT end, CMI is prominent and the lepromin skin test is positive by the Mitsuda reaction. Antibody titres are low. The infection is localised in this group and usually only a small number of skin lesions develop. Organisms infiltrate the nerves and the resulting CMI leads to fibrosis and thrombosis of the vasa nervorum that results in nerve lesions and anaesthesia. The histology of an active lesion shows tuberculoid granulomata, epithelioid cells and organisms. The lymphocyte transformation test *in vitro* is strongly positive.

At the LL end, CMI is weak but the antibody response is pronounced. The lepromin skin test is negative and the skin is heavily infiltrated with *M. leprae*. Untreated patients can suffer from bacteraemia, and bacilli are often present in large numbers in the spleen, liver and lymph nodes, especially those draining the skin. The paracortical area of the lymph nodes can be totally replaced by histiocytes containing acid-fast bacilli.

In contrast to *M. tuberculosis*, *M. leprae* cannot be grown in tissue culture.

2 Why has the patient developed erythema nodosum leprosum (ENL)?

There are often episodes of acute or chronic inflammation in leprosy, whether in association with treatment or not. The majority of reactions occur in patients receiving effective chemotherapy, and they do seem to be immunologically mediated. Over the course of a few days, the various leprosy lesions become inflamed, swollen and scaly, and new lesions can appear. Those lesions near nerves lead to local pain and further nerve damage. Patients feel ill and can have a high evening temperature. In severe ENL, the papules in the skin can ulcerate and this is frequently associated with joint pains and iridocyclitis.

The immunological changes may reflect the release of mycobacterial antigen, which in the presence of antibody forms immune complexes both locally and systemically causing the illness. A reduction in the load of bacilli allows a more marked CMI response to occur. This is seen in the inflammation in lesions which where previously inactive and which become swollen and inflamed. During the reaction, the lymphocyte transformation response to *M. leprae* rises and then falls when the reaction is successfully treated. The general histological appearance becomes more tuberculoid. A similar reaction can occur in peripheral nerves, and nerve destruction can develop unless prompt treatment is initiated.

Histologically, the lesions of ENL are similar to the Arthus reaction which is seen in typical Type III hypersensitivity, when antigen is injected into the skin of a subject with pre-existing IgG antibody. There is vasculitis and a polymorphonuclear infiltration superimposed on the resolving lepromatous granulomata.

3 What is the treatment for ENL?

In mild ENL, simple analgesics may be sufficient to control the symptoms. For severe ENL reactions, treatment is best managed in hospital. Corticosteroids in high doses are used in cases with severe neuritis, iridocyclitis or orchitis. Unfortunately, treatment may need to be prolonged and this brings the risk of steroid toxicity. Thalidomide also has strong anti-inflammatory activity and is the treatment of choice in acute ENL. The drug has the potential to induce a peripheral neuropathy but this has not yet been reported in ENL. Care must be taken if the patient is capable of child bearing.

4 Are there any genetic associations with the clinical response to *M. leprae*?

There are several extended haplotypes which are associated with hyper-responsiveness or susceptibility to a disease. In many situations HLA A-1, B-8, DR-3 is associated with hyper-responsiveness and this is also seen in leprosy. DR-3 especially is associated with increased T cell reactivity to *M. leprae* antigens in TT leprosy. There seems to be restriction of T-cell specificity to one mycobacterial protein (65 kDa) which indicates that the selection of epitopes is restricted by several HLA-DR genes.

MHC molecules class II , HLA-DQ1 and DR-2, have been found associated with the lepromatous form of the disease. Clinically, there is a strong association between DR3 negativity and lepromatous leprosy.

It is interesting that poorly degradable polysaccharide or glycolipid from bacilli may stay in the tissues for a long time after the organisms have been killed. These compounds, in particular, arabinomannan and lipoarabinomannan, can inhibit antigen processing for native antigens and therefore contribute to the anergy seen in the LL form of the disease.

■ CASE 35

Thiry-two-year-old Mrs Roberts was seen by a respiratory physician with a 2-month history of worsening lethargy, weakness and malaise and a weight loss of 3 kg. Recently, she had started sweating excessively at night and had felt flushed during the day. Over the past fortnight she had become mildly breathless on exertion and had developed a persistent dry cough. Her visit to the doctor was precipitated by the appearance of a red, hot and tender rash on her shins, upper arms and neck. She also complained of joint tenderness and itchy, inflamed eyes. Her only medical history of note was two normal pregnancies when aged 24 and 29 years. She had no history of tuberculosis or malignancy and was not currently taking any medication. A systems review did not reveal any further symptoms.

On examination, she had a temperature of 38.2°C but had no jaundice, anaemia, clubbing, cyanosis, oedema or lymphadenopathy. The doctor identified the red, hot and tender rash on her shins, upper arms and neck as erythema nodosum. The small joints of her hands were slightly tender, but there was no evidence of swelling. Conjunctivitis was present bilaterally but both optic fundi were normal. Her radial pulse was 78 beats/min and her blood pressure 125/75 mmHg. Her trachea was not deviated and she had normal chest expansion. Breath sounds were reduced bilaterally in all zones and were accompanied by widespread crackles. The apex beat was palpable and undeviated, and both heart sounds were present with no murmurs. Abdominal and neurological examinations were both unremarkable, with no hepatomegaly or splenomegaly. Results of investigations are shown in *Figure 35.1*.

A diagnosis of grade II sarcoidosis was made and Mrs Roberts was started on a course of oral prednisolone. At a follow-up appointment her symptoms were much improved and the erythema nodosum and conjunctivitis had cleared. Serum angiotensin converting enzyme (ACE) levels were decreased and the interstitial shadowing and lymphadenopathy on her chest X-ray had diminished. Within 12 months of presentation she had no remaining evidence of sarcoidosis and the steroids were discontinued.

QUESTIONS

1 What is the aetiology and pathogenesis of sarcoidosis?
2 How can sarcoidosis be classified clinically?
3 What is the cause of the hypercalcaemia and raised serum ACE levels?
4 What is the prognosis of sarcoidosis?

Investigation	Result *(normal range)*
Haemoglobin *(g/dl)*	12.1 *(11.5–16.0)*
White cell count *(x 10⁹/l)*	15.2 *(4.0–11.0)*
Neutrophils *(x 10⁹/l)*	8.2 *(2.0–7.5)*
Eosinophils *(x 10⁹/l)*	0.46 *(0.4–0.44)*
Total lymphocytes *(x 10⁹/l)*	1.2 *(1.6–3.5)*
Serum immunoglobulins	
IgG *(g/l)*	18.3 *(5.4–16.1)*
IgM *(g/l)*	2.7 *(0.5–1.9)*
IgA *(g/l)*	3.8 *(0.8–2.8)*
IgE *(IU/ml)*	51 *(3–150)*
Serum	
Sodium *(mmol/l)*	138 *(134–145)*
Potassium *(mmol/l)*	4.2 *(3.5–5.0)*
Chloride *(mmol/l)*	101 *(95–105)*
Calcium (total) *(mmol/l)*	2.82 *(2.12–2.65)*
Phosphate *(mmol/l)*	1.25 *(0.8–1.45)*
Creatinine *(μmol/l)*	101 *(70–150)*
Urea *(mmol/l)*	3.4 *(2.5–6.7)*
ESR	49 mm/hr
Serum angiotensin converting enzyme *(IU/l)*	123 *(25–69)*
Mantoux test	
1 tuberculin units	Negative
10 tuberculin units	Negative
Kveim test	Positive
Chest X-ray	Bilateral hilar lymphadenopathy. Bilateral mid-zone interstitial shadowing
Abdominal X-ray	Normal
Liver biopsy	Multiple epithelioid granulomas
Bronchoalveolar lavage (BAL)	Lymphocytic alveolitis CD4⁺:CD8⁺ = 10:1
Lung function tests	Decreased FVC Decreased FEV1 Normal ratio

Fig. 35.1 Results of investigations.

■ **CASE 35** pp. 349–352

ANSWERS

1 What is the aetiology and pathogenesis of sarcoidosis?

Sarcoidosis can be defined as a multisystem disorder characterised by the development of non-caseating, epithelioid granulomas. The incidence in the UK is around 20/100 000, with the highest rate found in Irish immigrants and those of West Indian origin (150–180/100 000). The aetiology of the disease is unknown with mycobacteria, viruses, fungi and agents such as beryllium putatively suggested as causal factors. Patients with sarcoidosis are more frequently mycobacteria positive than controls, but the evidence is equivocal. Some authors believe that sarcoidosis is not a single disease entity but a syndrome caused by a variety of agents.

A typical sarcoid lesion consists of well defined granulomata of epithelioid cells surrounded by a border of lymphocytes, mainly CD4$^+$. Giant multinucleate cells are also occasionally seen. There is a paucity of CD4$^+$ cells in the peripheral blood of sarcoid patients, probably because of recruitment into the granulomas. In common with the lesions found in tuberculosis, sarcoid granulomas consist of epithelioid cells derived from locally recruited macrophages and blood-borne monocytes. Unlike TB, however, the lesions do not caseate.

It is widely believed that an abnormality of the T helper/suppressor cell balance plays a role in the pathogenesis of sarcoidosis, although it is not known whether an increase in the former or a decrease in the latter is responsible. Analysis of BAL specimens from sarcoid patients has demonstrated a diminution of αβ receptors on pulmonary T cells despite an increase in T-cell receptor (TCR) messenger RNA. The implication for T-cell regulation remains unclear. IL-2 receptor levels in serum and on pulmonary macrophages and monocytes are increased in active disease, suggesting a pivotal role for IL-2. IL-1, IL-6 and TNFα are also likely to play a part in the activation of macrophages and endothelial cells as well as in lymphocyte recruitment. This has been demonstrated by assaying the levels of these mediators, which correlate with disease activity as measured by BAL lymphocyte numbers.

Active pulmonary lesions also contain large quantities of B lymphocytes. The secretion of IL-2 and IL-4 by T cells found in sarcoidosis lesions drives B cell proliferation, and may be responsible for the hypergammaglobulinaemia which is frequently found in these patients.

2 How can sarcoidosis be classified clinically?

Sarcoidosis can affect almost any organ or tissue of the body. The most common site is the lungs, with lesions found in 85% of cases. An abnormal routine chest X-ray often leads to the initial diagnosis in the absence of symptoms. Erythema nodosum occurs in 20–30% of cases, with skin lesions in 15% and bone cysts in 5%. Eye involvement, which is found in up to a quarter of subjects, may cause blindness. Lymphadenopathy and enlargement of salivary glands are also common.

Thoracic sarcoid can be classified by radiography into three stages. Half of all patients present with stage I disease, hilar lymphadenopathy. Most are asymptomatic although some have a dry cough and mild chest pain. Stage II, with both hilar lymphadenopathy and parenchymal infiltrates, is found in 30% of patients. A greater percentage of these patients are symptomatic than those with stage I disease, and a restrictive lung defect may be demonstrated by spirometry. Stage III disease is characterised by pulmonary fibrosis and associated breathlessness, which may progress to pulmonary hypertension.

3 What is the cause of the hypercalcaemia and raised serum ACE levels?

Hypercalcaemia is present in 10–50% of patients during the active phase of the disease. This is caused by an increased conversion of 2,5-hydroxycholecalciferol to 1,25-dihydroxycholecalciferol (calcitriol) by pulmonary macrophages. Calcitriol promotes the intestinal absorption of calcium and phosphate and therefore raises the serum calcium concentration. Serum ACE, which is similarly produced by sarcoid macrophages, correlates with disease activity as measured by BAL lymphocyte numbers. The test is not diagnostic as raised levels may be found in patients without sarcoidosis.

4 What is the prognosis of sarcoidosis?

In over half of all patients with thoracic sarcoidosis, the disease resolves within 2 years without treatment. A further quarter of cases will resolve with oral corticosteroid treatment. In over 90% of those with stage I sarcoid, the disease resolves within 2 years, with this figure dropping to 50% in the stage II group. Only 30% of those with stage III disease respond to steroids. Treatment is advised in all patients with stage II and III disease associated with high serum ACE levels. Other indications include involvement of the eyes, heart, nervous system and salivary glands and the presence of hypercalcaemia or breathlessness.

CASE 36

Mrs Nakrani, a 28-year-old housewife, presented to her GP with a 1-week history of abdominal pain. She described her symptoms as a discomfort that spread across her abdomen. The discomfort was associated with intermittent colicky pain which caused her to double over at times. She also reported a 2-day history of loose stools and an excess of flatus. She had not passed any blood in her stools. Her GP could only elicit some mild, diffuse abdominal tenderness, with no masses and a normal rectal examination. A diagnosis of gastroenteritis was made, and Mrs Nakrani was advised to stay at home until her symptoms settled.

Mrs Nakrani became increasingly unwell at home. Her abdominal pains intensified, and she had regular bouts of colic, some of which woke her up. Her diarrhoea became profuse and bloody, and she visited the toilet up to 12 times a day and several times at night. She also developed sore areas around her anus, several painful mouth ulcers, and a tender rash on the front of both her calves. Her appetite fell, and she became increasingly dehydrated. Her husband decided to take her to the local Accident & Emergency department.

On arrival at hospital, Mrs Nakrani looked unwell. She was clinically dehydrated with a blood pressure of 110/75 mmHg lying and 85/60 mmHg standing. She also had a mild tachycardia of 95 beats/min. She had no peripheral oedema, and had no finger clubbing. The remainder of her cardiovascular and respiratory examinations were unremarkable. She had two, small aphthous mouth ulcers on her hard palate. Her abdomen was soft, with widespread tenderness. Her right iliac fossa was particularly tender, although no mass was palpable. Her bowel sounds were elevated, but not high pitched or 'tinkly'. A rectal examination showed a small area of perianal ulceration with soft, bloody stool on the glove. The rash on her legs consisted of raised, red macules which were classical for erythema nodosum. The results of investigations are shown in *Figure 36.1*.

A flexible sigmoidoscopy was performed which showed multiple areas of ulceration with some perianal disease. Biopsies were performed which demonstrated classical Crohn's disease. A barium follow through was carried out to determine the extent of her Crohn's disease. Several small areas of ulceration were seen in her ileum, although none were affecting the terminal region and there was no evidence of stricturing.

Mrs Nakrani was started on a course of mesalazine tablets and oral steroids. A dietician advised an elemental diet, and oral iron therapy was started for her mild iron deficiency anaemia. Mrs Nakrani's symptoms settled over a period of 10 days, and she was discharged on her elemental diet, to continue for 1 month, and a continuing course of mesalazine. Foods were re-introduced one at a time into her diet. Those that caused reactions were voided.

QUESTIONS

1 What is the histopathology of Crohn's disease?
2 What is the pathogenesis of Crohn's disease?
3 What part do elemental diets play in managing acute exacerbations of Crohn's disease?

Investigation	Result (normal range)
Haemoglobin (g/dl)	10.3 (11.5–16.0)
MCV (fl)	77.2
White cell count (x 10⁹/l)	13.2 (4.0–11.0)
Neutrophil count (x 10⁹/l)	9.5 (2.0–7.5)
Platelet count (x 10⁹/l)	490 (150–400)
Serum	
Sodium (mmol/l)	132 (134–145)
Potassium (mmol/l)	3.2 (3.5–5.0)
Urea (mmol/l)	7.5 (2.5–6.7)
Creatinine (mmol/l)	105 (70–150)
Liver function tests	
Alanine transaminase (IU/ml)	52 (5–35)
Alkaline phosphatase (IU/l)	70 (30–300)
Serum bilirubin (μmol/l)	18 (3–17)
Serum albumin (g/l)	31 (35–50)
ESR	59 mm/hr (<20)
C reactive protein	32 (<5)
Mantoux test	Positive, 5 mm erythema and induration
Chest X-ray	Normal
Abdominal X-ray	Multiple short regions of distended bowel loops

Fig. 36.1 Results of investigations.

■ **CASE 36** p. 351

ANSWERS

1 What is the histopathology of Crohn's disease?

Crohn's disease can affect any part of the gastrointestinal tract from the mouth to the anus. The most common site is the terminal ileum, with inherent implications for the absorption of nutrients. Macroscopically, the gut wall becomes thickened, producing a narrowing of the bowel lumen. Stricturing may be severe and can cause proximal dilation. The intestinal mucosa becomes ulcerated, with intervening oedematous areas producing a 'cobblestone' appearance. Regional lymph nodes may also become involved in the inflammatory process. Deep fissures may traverse the gut wall leading to abscess formation.

Histologically, all layers of the bowel wall are affected by an inflammatory infiltrate. The classical feature, as described by Crohn and his colleagues, is the presence of non-caseating epithelioid granulomas, which may lead to crypt destruction. Obstruction of the lymphatics of the infiltrate is likely to explain the mucosal oedema. Chronic inflammatory infiltrates, fibrosis and gastric type metaplasia may occur.

Immunologically, the leucocyte infiltrate consists of lymphocytes, plasma cells and eosinophils. The cells express high levels of activation markers such as the IL-2 receptor, while epithelial cells have increased major histocompatibility complex II expression.

2 What is the pathogenesis of Chron's disease?

Crohn's disease has a prevalence of approximately 50/100 000, with four new cases/100 000 of the population in a year. The incidence appears to be rising. It is very uncommon in Afrocaribbeans. The disease was first characterised by Dr B Crohn in New York in the early 1930s. He was the first worker to confirm earlier suspicions of granulomatous disorders in which mycobacteria were not involved. The original classification described a 'terminal ileitis', but when it became clear that any part of the gut could be involved, the term 'regional enteritis' was adopted.

The pathogenesis of Crohn's disease remains elusive. As with all diseases a mixture of genetics and environment appear to be responsible. Some 10% of patients with the disease have a relative with inflammatory bowel disease, although most have ulcerative colitis rather than Crohn's disease. No prominent HLA associations exist. It is worthy of note that Crohn's is associated with ankylosing spondylitis although, interestingly, most cases are HLA-B27 negative. A low fibre and high refined sugar diet appears to be associated with an increased risk of Crohn's disease. Controlled trials have now shown the benefit of identifying and eliminating culprit foods in the long term management of this condition. Infectious agents have also been suggested to cause the inflammatory process, but firm evidence is lacking. Many workers in this field believe that such an aetiology is likely however, with a slow growing mycobacteria or mycobacteria-like organism hypothesised or even measles.

3 What part do elemental diets play in managing acute exacerbations of Chron's disease?

It was first noted in the 1970s that the use of parenteral nutrition could prevent some patients with inflammatory bowel disease requiring surgical intervention. At this stage it was believed that a period of 'bowel rest' explained this phenomenon. However, a controlled trial of total parenteral nutrition versus total enteral nutrition conducted in 1988 showed similar short-term remission and long-term outcome measures. This dispelled the myth that 'bowel rest' was the critical factor in improving outcome. Total parenteral nutrition is not now regarded as a primary treatment of uncomplicated but active Crohn's disease.

Elemental diets are a mixture of glucose, amino acids, vitamins, minerals, trace elements and a small quantity of fat. The mixture is absorbed without the aid of pancreatic enzymes. Importantly, it is unlikely that elemental diets contain any antigenic potential unlike peptide (oligomeric) based diets which may still have such potential. Patients produce a solution of the mixture with water, which they take to the exclusion of their normal diet for a period of weeks. Complicance is certainly an issue because of the unpalatable nature of the diet.

Remission rates in active Crohn's disease with elemental diet treatment are at least as comparable as reducing regimens of corticosteroids. In some trials, the rate was superior. In severe active disease, the two therapies can of course be used in combination. Particular areas of use include the paediatric setting, where growth retardation is a problem with acute Crohn's disease. Elemental diets not only improve the patient's nutritional status, but reduce the need for corticosteroid treatment, with its inherent growth retardation properties. Pregnancy is another area where steroid independence is of importance.

Although the mechanism of action of elemental diets is not understood, many believe that the reduction of food antigen load is of importance in reducing mucosal inflammation. Decreased gut permeability to antigens may also play a role.

CASE 37

Forty-year-old Mrs Chari was seen in Accident & Emergency after several episodes of painless haematuria. On direct questioning she complained of worsening malaise and increasing generalised oedema over the previous 2 weeks. She also noted that despite a high fluid intake she was passing urine far less frequently than normal. She had no medical history of note and had never suffered from diabetes, hypertension or connective tissue disease. A systems review revealed a recent history of dizziness, but no further symptoms.

On examination, Mrs Chari was clinically anaemic and had generalised pitting oedema. Her temperature was 38.2°C, and her blood pressure was 155/110 mmHg. A respiratory examination did not reveal any basal crepitations. The apex beat was palpable and undeviated but her jugular venous pulse was not visible. Both heart sounds were present and there were no murmurs. Abdominal examination did not reveal any palpable masses or hepatosplenomegaly. A neurological assessment demonstrated a mild degree of disorientation but no other abnormalities. Results of investigations are shown in *Figure 37.1*.

A diagnosis of idiopathic crescentic (rapidly progressive) glomerulonephritis was made. Despite the use of antihypertensive agents, corticosteroids and azathioprine, Mrs Chari's renal function deteriorated and end-stage renal failure was diagnosed. Regular haemodialysis was commenced and Mrs Chari was tissue typed for major histocompatibility antigens (MHC) using anti-HLA antibodies in preparation for a possible renal transplant. Her profile was found to be HLA -A10, -A28, -B7, -Bw52, -Cw2, -Cw6, -DR2, -DRw10, with blood group B positive. A suitable cadaveric kidney was found from a donor of HLA type -A9, -A11, -B7, -B17, -Cw2, -Cw8, -DR2, -DR4, and the same blood group. A cross-match of Mrs Chari's serum with donor lymphocytes was also satisfactory.

Transplantation was combined with the triple immunosuppressive regimen of prednisolone, cyclosporin A, and azathioprine to aid acceptance of the graft. Serum creatinine and urea levels fell postoperatively and hourly urine output from the graft was satisfactory. Her blood pressure dropped to 140/90 mmHg.

Ten days following the transplant Mrs Chari developed a fever and was noted to be lethargic. On examination, she had peripheral oedema and her blood pressure was 145/110 mmHg. Her urine output had dropped to 25 ml/hr and she was tender in the region of the graft. As there was no evidence of post-renal obstruction, infection, hypovolaemia or cyclosporin toxicity, a percutaneous renal biopsy was carried out. Histological analysis demonstrated significant interstitial mononuclear cell infiltration and severe tubulitis. A diagnosis of acute grade II rejection was made and Mrs Chari was prescribed parenteral methylprednisolone. This failed to improve her renal function and OKT3 (an anti-lymphocyte monoclonal antibody preparation specific for T-cell CD3) was administered. This improved her renal function and she was eventually discharged on cyclosporin A.

QUESTIONS

1 What types of rejection syndromes exist?
2 What factors are important in matching donor to recipient in renal transplantation?

Investigation	Result *(normal range)*
Haemoglobin *(g/dl)*	10.0 *(11.5–16.0)*
White cell count *(x 10⁹/l)*	13.2 *(4.0–11.0)*
Serum	
Sodium *(mmol/l)*	149 *(134–145)*
Potassium *(mmol/l)*	5.5 *(3.5–5.0)*
Chloride *(mmol/l)*	109 *(95–105)*
Creatinine *(µmol/l)*	410 *(70–150)*
Urea *(mmol/l)*	17.1 *(2.5–6.7)*
Serum albumin *(g/l)*	28 *(35–50)*
ESR	98 mm/hr
Urine	
Visual inspection	Macroscopic haematuria
Microscopy	~5 white cells/ml
	Red cells ++
	Granular casts
Culture	<10⁴ mixed organisms/ml
24 hr protein loss	2.2 g
Abdominal X-ray	Normal
Renal biopsy	Proliferation of glomerular, endothelial and mesangial cells. Variable polymorph infiltrate. Crescent formation in part of the sample
Serum complement	
C3 *(g/l)*	0.98 *(0.75–1.65)*
C4 *(g/l)*	0.41 *(0.20–0.65)*
ANA	Negative
Anti-GBM antibodies	Negative
Anti-streptococcal antibodies	
Streptolysin O (ASO)	Negative
DNase B	Negative
Hyaluronidase	Negative

Fig. 37.1 Results of investigations.

■ CASE 37   p. 323, Chapter 27

ANSWERS

1 What types of rejection syndromes exist?

Renal transplant rejection is classified according to the timing of the episode. Hyperacute rejection occurs minutes to hours following transplantation. It arises when the graft recipient has antibodies to either MHC class I or ABO blood group antigens, both of which are expressed on the renal epithelium. Recipient pre-sensitisation may occur following blood transfusions, previous transplantation or pregnancy. Complement activation causes recruitment of lymphocytes and platelets into the graft which rapidly becomes thrombosed and infarcted. Removal of the kidney is inevitable. This kind of rejection is now rarely seen due to effective donor/recipient cross-matching.

Accelerated rejection occurs 3–5 days following transplantation. Presensitised cytotoxic T lymphocytes or non-complement-binding antibodies may be responsible. The latter mediate an antibody-dependent, cell-mediated, cytotoxic reaction against the graft by binding to Fc receptors. Vascular endothelium is often targeted because it expresses MHC I and II molecules. Histologically the graft is oedematous and infiltrated with mononuclear cells. Immunosuppressive agents may save the graft but there is an increased risk of eventual failure.

Acute rejection, which takes place 7 days to 3 months following transplantation, accounts for 85% of all rejection episodes. Cellular rejection is a CD8+ T cell mediated (type IV) phenomenon characterised histologically by oedema and cellular infiltration. In addition, varying degrees of vascular rejection are present, initiated by IgG or IgM antibodies to vascular wall components (a Type II reaction). The severity of the rejection episode is graded by these vascular changes as mild (grade I), moderate (grade II) or severe (grade III). Grafts may be saved with high dose methylprednisolone, or, in resistant cases, by OKT3 or antithymocyte globulin (ATG) therapy.

Chronic rejection presents insidiously 3 months to years after transplantation and appears to be an immune complex mediated phenomenon. Vascular changes include platelet and fibrin deposition with intimal proliferation. In the glomeruli, there is often mesangial hyperplasia and focal basement membrane thickening. Immunosuppressive treatment is ineffective, and the graft is usually lost.

2 What factors are important in matching donor to recipient in renal transplantation?

Two groups of antigens are important in renal transplantation: the ABO blood group system and the human leukocyte antigens (HLAs). When a donor kidney is sought it must first meet the criterion of ABO compatibility with the recipient. As with a blood transfusion a group O kidney could be given to any recipient. A degree of matching at the HLA locus, found on chromosome 6, is also of benefit.

The HLA locus contains three classes of genes, I, II and III (*Fig. 37.2*). The HLA class I genes A, B and C encode the major histocompatibility class I antigens (MHC I) which present endogenous peptides to CD8+ T cells. The HLA class II genes DP, DQ and DR encode the MHC II antigens which present exogenously derived peptides to CD4+ T cells. The class III locus is a diverse group which includes genes for alternative pathway complement components and TNFα and β.

The most widely used test for the identification of HLA antigens is the microlymphocytotoxicity test. Lymphocytes from the individual to be tested are incubated with sera containing antibodies to known HLA haplotypes. Cell death indicates a positive result. The principle of this procedure is also used following donor/recipient HLA matching. Donor lymphocytes are incubated with recipient serum to detect antibodies to MHC I and II molecules. The presence of antibodies to MHC I may preclude the use of the graft.

The issue of HLA matching in renal transplantation is controversial. Grafts between HLA-identical siblings have the longest survival whereas a complete mismatch is associated with poor survival. Recent data suggest that graft survival is not significantly influenced by the degree of mismatch. For example, the survival time for a graft HLA mismatched by one haplotype is not significantly different from one mismatched by 4 haplotypes. In practice HLA matching is carried out as far as possible with the focus on the MHC II molecules.

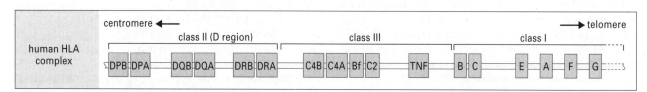

Fig. 37.2 Organisation of the human major histocompatibility complex genes.

CASE 38

Miss Jacob, a 30-year-old Caribbean woman, had been visiting her doctor for some time with aches and pains in her joints. The year before, following a flight from the Caribbean, she developed a severe pain in her left leg and was found to have a deep vein thrombosis. The cause of the venous thrombosis was thought to be venous stasis because of the long plane flight and she was treated with anticoagulants. She then developed other symptoms such as headache, occasional bouts of acute abdominal pain – all this being associated with lethargy, occasional fever and some loss of weight.

She had just returned from holiday when she was sent to the rheumatologist who found that she had a rash on her face and some patchy hair loss on her scalp. Her joints were tender but not very swollen. Her muscles ached and she complained of chest pain. The results of investigations are shown in *Figure 38.1*.

A diagnosis of systemic lupus erythematosus (SLE) was made. Miss Jacob was treated in the first instance with chloroquine, an antimalarial, for the rash on her face and chest. She was strongly advised to have an examination of her eyes every 6 months because of the potential side effects of the chloroquine treatment.

At a follow-up appointment, she was found to have pain in the calf of her leg, and further information of her medical history was obtained. Three years previously she had suffered a spontaneous

abortion. Although not commonly associated with SLE, she was then diagnosed as having the antiphospholipid syndrome and treated with anticoagulants. Her renal function showed an elevated serum creatinine with red cells and protein in her urine. This prompted a renal biopsy which gave the histological picture of diffuse proliferative lupus nephritis. She was then treated with oral corticosteroids, immunosuppressants and an antihypertensive drug.

Ten years later, she was still attending the clinic and still required treatment.

QUESTIONS

1 What information can be obtained from autoantibody tests in patients with SLE?
2 What is the immunopathological mechanism leading to the glomerulonephritis?
3 What are the main characteristics of the antiphospholipid syndrome (APS)?
4 Is SLE a classic autoimmune disease?

Investigations	Results *(normal range)*
Haemoglobin *(g/dl)*	10.3 *(11.5–16.0)*
Blood film	Normocytic, normochromic red cells
White cell count *(x 10⁹/l)*	3.4 *(4.0–11.0)*
Haemoglobin electrophoresis	No evidence of thalassaemia or sickle cell disease
C reactive protein *(mg/l)*	45 *(<5)*
ESR	52 mm/hr
DAT	Positive
Autoantibodies	
Rheumatoid factor	Negative
ANA	Positive, titre 1:640
dsDNA binding activity	>80%
Anti-RNA	Positive
Anti-histone	Positive
Anti-cardiolipin	Positive
Serum	
C3 *(g/l)*	0.45 *(0.75–1.65)*
C4 *(g/l)*	0.12 *(0.20–0.65)*
Skin biopsy from unaffected area	Deposition of complement and IgG at dermo-epidermal junction. Positive lupus 'band' test

Fig. 38.1 Results of investigations.

■ CASE 38   pp. 325–326, 329, 332, 367–369, 373

ANSWERS

1   What information can be obtained from autoantibody tests in patients with SLE?

The main autoantibodies in patients with SLE are directed against nucleic acids and proteins concerned with intracellular transcription and translation. The screening test for antinuclear antibodies (ANA) is by indirect immunofluorescence on tissue sections or Hep 2 cells. Over 95% of patients with SLE have ANA. Autoantibodies are found directed against several cell components: nucleic acid and histones, ribonucleoproteins (RNP), phospholipids and membrane antigens.

The most characteristic antibody in SLE is that to DNA, especially double stranded DNA (dsDNA). Antibodies to single stranded DNA (ssDNA) are less specific and can be found in other conditions. Antibodies directed against 'extractable nuclear proteins' were originally designated by the initials of the patients in whom they were first found, e.g. Sm for Smith. Antibody to Sm is found in a variable proportion of SLE patients; in 5% of whites and 25% of blacks and Chinese. Two common autoantibodies recognise Ro and La particles which were originally identified as RNP species but have also been found in the nucleus.

Many autoantibodies react with cell surfaces and are thought to be the cause of leucopaenia, thrombocytopaenia and haemolytic anaemia found in SLE.

2   What is the immunopathological mechanism leading to glomerulonephritis?

SLE is one of the multisystem vasculitides. Renal involvement is common but treatable. Immune complex deposition in the kidney makes a causal role for autoantibodies and complement very likely. Renal involvement correlates with low levels of C3 and C4 suggesting classical pathway activation. One of the problems is that 'antigen' in the form of DNA has not been found as a component in circulating immune complexes from patients with SLE. However, anti dsDNA and antiidiotype antibodies can be eluted from kidney tissue confirming that immune complex deposition does occur in the organ. Free DNA can fix to glomeruli in mice which could then react with ANA.

It is likely that multiple antigen–antibody systems operate in SLE and the immune complexes involved may differ from patient to patient. The location of the deposits governs the type of pathology seen in the kidney. The WHO classification is based on the pathology of the glomerular lesions and the majority of patients fall into one of the diagnostic groups.

- Class I; normal kidneys.
- Class II; mesangial changes.
- Class III; focal and segmental proliferative glomerulonephritis and/or necrotising glomerulonephritis.
- Class IV; diffuse proliferative and necrotising glomerulonephritis.
- Class V; membranous glomerulonephritis.

3   What are the main characteristics of the antiphospholipid syndrome (APS)?

Some patients with SLE have a false positive test for syphilis, a positive Wassermann reaction. Another antiphospholipid antibody (aPL), known as the 'lupus anticoagulant', is present in a subgroup of SLE patients. This antibody is associated with increased coagulation and recurrent thrombosis *in vivo* although it delays clotting time *in vitro*. It inhibits coagulation by interfering with the binding of vitamin K dependent proteins to the phospholipid component of the prothrombin activator complex.

The increased thrombosis seen in patients may be due to platelet activation or binding to endothelium and inhibition of prostacyclin release. Recurrent spontaneous abortion is a notable feature of the syndrome. In mice with APS, there is an increased rate of foetal absorption, and live foetuses and placentae are smaller than those seen in control animals.

The vessels affected by thrombosis can be venous or arterial. The major features are deep vein thrombosis, strokes, transient ischaemic attacks, multi-infarct dementia and, commonly, thrombocytopaenia. Minor features are leg ulcers, livedo reticularis and haemolytic anaemia. Less common presentations can be migraine, labile hypertension, osteonecrosis and the Guillain–Barré syndrome.

4   Is SLE a classic autoimmune disease?

SLE is certainly the classical example of non-organ specific autoimmunity and autoantibodies are the most striking feature of the disease. What is not certain is whether the antibodies actually cause the syndrome. Transfusion of serum with high titres of ANA does not cause SLE.

As with many other autoimmune diseases, the presence of autoantibodies is a marker of the condition, a prerequisite for disease but not sufficient to cause the lesions.

There are many theories as to the aetiology of SLE but none of them completely explains the disease. If the ability to clear immune complexes is reduced, there could be a stimulation of autoimmunity by autoantigens. Immune complex clearance is less in subjects with null genes for C4, C1q and C2, and this could represent a susceptibility factor.

Polyclonal activation of B cells would lead to proliferation of all antibody producing cells including those producing autoantibodies. Studies in human lupus suggest that the autoantibody response is specific and is driven by antigen with no polyclonal activation of B cells. A disturbance of the idiotypic-antiidiotypic network could stimulate autoantibody production. Antiidiotypic antibodies to anti-DNA antibodies have been found, but usually in patients with inactive disease. Although immunisation with a monoclonal antiidiotypic antibody can suppress the idiotype transiently, it was soon overcome with large amounts of anti-dsDNA antibodies. A further possibility, the breaking of tolerance through molecular mimicry by microbial antigens, has not been shown in the human variant of the disease.

■ CASE 39

Forty-five-year-old Mrs Smith visited her doctor after noticing a painless swelling at the front of her neck. On questioning she said that it had taken 2–3 years to reach its present size. She was otherwise in good health.

On examination Mrs Smith's thyroid was found to be diffusely enlarged and firm, the enlargement including the isthmus of the gland producing a 'butterfly' appearance. Apart from the lump in her neck she felt quite well. In particular she did not feel tired or lethargic. Measurement of serum T3, T4, and thyroid stimulating hormone (TSH) using specific radioimmunoassays produced results within the normal ranges, demonstrating that Mrs Smith had normal thyroid function. Tests for autoantibodies were positive in that she had significant levels of antithyroglobulin and antithyroid microsomal antibodies (antithyroid peroxidase; anti-TPO).

She continued to remain well but her doctor decided to keep her under supervision. Over the next 3–4 years she did begin to feel more tired and she preferred to sleep in the armchair when she got home instead of being the hive of activity that was her previous habit. She also became slower in her movements and her husband noted that her memory had deteriorated and that her actions were clumsy. Her weight increased and all her relatives noticed that her voice had become more husky. She also had dry skin and a 'puffy' face. She returned to her doctor for further evaluation.

On examination her radial pulse was 55 beats/min. Her goitre had not increased in size. There was some thinning of her hair and the outer border of her eyebrows had disappeared. Her joints ached, she had some tingling in her fingers and when the doctor tested her reflexes there was delayed relaxation. Results of investigations are shown in *Figure 39.1*. Her thyroid autoantibodies were elevated compared with her initial results. Mrs Smith was diagnosed as having Hashimoto's thyroiditis (HT).

On discussing her family history she remembered a first degree relative with pernicious anaemia.

She started treatment with a low dose of T4 which was increased slowly over the next few months. Her TSH was used as a monitor of response to treatment and it returned to normal levels when her T4 dose reached 150 µg daily. All her previous symptoms disappeared, including her aching joints and the tingling in her fingers. She also regained all her previous vim and vigour.

QUESTIONS

1 Is there a genetic predisposition to autoimmune disease?
2 What are the mechanisms of immunological damage to the thyroid?
3 Does the presence of autoantibodies signify the presence of disease?
4 What are the autoantigens in Hashimoto's thyroiditis?

Investigation	Result (normal range)
Haemoglobin (g/dl)	14.3 (11.5–16.0)
White cell count (x 10⁹/l)	6.4 (4.0–11.0)
Lymphocytes (x 10⁹/l)	2.1 (1.6–3.5)
Serum	
Urea (mmol/l)	3.2 (2.5–6.7)
Sodium (mmol/l)	141 (134–145)
Potassium (mmol/l)	4.0 (3.5–5.0)
Chloride (mmol/l)	101 (95–105)
Serum free T4 (pmol/l)	6.8 (9–22)
Serum free T3 (nmol/l)	0.8 (1.2–3.0)
TSH (mU/l)	16.4 (0.5–5.7)
Autoantibodies	
Thyroglobulin	1:640
Thyroid microsomes	1:32 000
Gastric parietal cells	1:320
ANA	Negative

Fig. 39.1 Results of investigations.

■ CASE 39   pp. 331–332

ANSWERS

1 Is there a genetic predisposition to autoimmune disease?

There is certainly a greater incidence of autoantibodies in family members of patients with HT than in the normal population. In addition, there is a link between HT and pernicious anaemia, where anti-parietal cell and anti-intrinsic factor antibodies lead to the malabsorption of vitamin B12. Patients with HT have a greater incidence of pernicious anaemia than controls and the reverse is also true; patients with pernicious anaemia have a greater incidence of HT. This evidence from family studies does point to a genetic predisposition.

Initial studies suggested that there was an HLA association of HLA-DR5 with HT and HLA-DR3 with primary myxoedema. However, this is not always the case because in some populations HLA-DR3 is linked with HT. If thyroid tissue from an HT patient is examined by polymerase chain reaction, both DQA1*0301 (in linkage disequilibrium with HLA-DR4) and DQB1*0201 (in linkage disequilibrium with HLA-DR3) are increased, giving similar relative risks.

The populations that have been studied are ethnically diverse and it is not surprising that differences in HLA associations are found. Recent studies from Japan have found no HLA association with HT.

The situation can be summarised by saying that HLA encoded genes do not confer strong susceptibility to HT, and there is considerable population variation in HLA association. This suggests that there are significant endogenous or exogenous factors determining susceptibility.

2 What are the mechanisms of immunological damage to the thyroid?

As with many autoimmune diseases there can be a number of damaging mechanisms producing disease in the gland. The hallmark of HT is the presence of circulating autoantibodies that can cause damage through Type II hypersensitivity reactions. However, thyroglobulin antibodies do not fix complement, but antibodies to thyroid peroxidase (TPOa) can activate the complement pathway. There may be other unspecified autoantibodies that can also fix complement. Suggestive of Type II hypersensitivity mechanisms is the finding of complement on the surface of the thyroid cell and, more recently the production of membrane attack complexes at the site of the thyroid follicles in HT. When a thyroid cell has been attacked by complement there will also be a release of PGE_2, IL-1 and IL-6 as well as reactive oxygen intermediates. These can cause direct injury to the thyrocyte and lead to further lymphocyte infiltration and activation.

The classic autoantibody in HT may also cause damage by binding to the surface of the thyroid cell, allowing natural killer cells to bind through Fc receptor binding – antibody dependent cell cytotoxicity (ADCC). This mechanism can be shown *in vitro* using normal thyroid cells, autoantibody and normal lymphocytes as effector cells.

3 Does the presence of autoantibodies signify the presence of disease?

It does seem that the prevalence of HT is increasing. It may be that the assay systems have become more sensitive, or that the disease is indeed more common. What is clear is that there is a significant number of people who are asymptomatic who have detectable levels of antithyroglobulin antibodies (TGa) in their circulation. Even in the young age group (18–24 years) the prevalence of TGa is 10%, while in an older cohort (55–64 years) it is 30%. On long-term follow-up, it has been shown that patients can have antibodies for many years without progressing to clinical HT.

One possibility is that the thyroglobulin from patients with HT is different to that of normal individuals and that explains the progression to disease. However, no differences have been found in the thyroglobulin structure itself, although the effect of iodination on immunogenicity is not clear.

Perhaps the best predictor for disease is a strong family history of HT.

4 What are the autoantigens in HT?

The concept of organ-specific autoimmune disease was first introduced by Roitt, Doniach and Campbell more than 30 years ago. They were able to show TGa in the sera of HT patients using a very simple agar precipitation technique.

Thyroglobulin (660 kDa) may have up to seven linear epitopes that are recognised by TGa, although the profile of the response in individual patients is very varied. Thyroglobulin is expressed on the surface of the thyroid cell but is difficult to detect. The affinity of TGa for the antigen varies and is likely to vary in any case during the course of the disease.

The second autoantigen was originally the thyroid microsomal antigen now characterised as TPO. This is a membrane bound protein of 100–105 kDa. Various sites have been defined on the molecule, with at least six B-cell epitopes on the native molecule as well as one or two linear epitopes.

In some patients there are antibodies that cross-react with both thyroglobulin and TPO. The functional activity of these antibodies is not known.

Probably the most important 'antigen' from the point of view of thyroid function is the thyroid stimulating hormone receptor (TSH-R). Antibodies against this receptor may act in a similar manner to TSH and stimulate the gland, as is seen in Graves' disease, or block the action of the receptor and contribute to hypothyroidism. Anti-TSH-R antibodies are present in almost all patients with Graves' disease. Unlike TGa, which are not highly predictive for thyroiditis, the presence of anti-TSH-R antibodies makes the subsequent development of Graves' disease highly likely.

CASE 40

When Mrs Booth went for her annual check-up at the age of 52 she was found to be fit but to have a raised alkaline phosphatase. She had no cough in spite of smoking 40 cigarettes a day. Other routine investigations at the time showed nothing untoward and her chest X-ray was clear. Over the next few years, her alkaline phosphatase levels increased and she showed a slight but significant increase in the level of aspartate transaminase and alanine transaminase. She then went to her doctor with a number of complaints which were rather vague in nature. She was still smoking 40 cigarettes a day. Her bowels were not quite right and she had some diarrhoea, which was very unusual for her. She thought that she had been bitten by midges because of occasional itching, and she had more aches and pains than she had ever had before. She also complained of a dry mouth and had to keep on taking sips of water.

The doctor examined her and did not find anything strikingly abnormal. There were no palpable lymph nodes, and no abnormality on examination of her chest or heart. The preliminary blood tests taken at that time are shown in *Figure 40.1*.

He noticed the raised bilirubin level and the tests for hepatitis B surface antigen which were negative. Mrs Booth later developed a palpable spleen and moderate ascites. Several diagnoses were considered when no evidence of neoplastic disease was found.

She was referred to a surgeon who found an enlarged liver and wondered if she had a small pleural effusion. A further chest X-ray was normal. The surgeon still felt that secondary deposits from carcinoma of the bronchus was likely but bronchoscopy was clear and no abnormal cells were seen on bronchial lavage. Further investigations by the surgeon showed a raised IgM and eventually autoantibodies were measured. She was found to have high titres of antimitochondrial antibodies (AMA). Liver biopsy confirmed the diagnosis of primary biliary cirrhosis (PBC).

QUESTIONS

1 What is the autoantigen in PBC?
2 What is thought to be the mechanism of damage to the liver?
3 What are the associated syndromes in patients with PBC?
4 What treatment can be given to patients with PBC?

Investigation	Result *(normal range)*
Haemoglobin *(g/dl)*	12.3 *(11.5–16.0)*
White cell count *(x 10⁹/l)*	7.3 *(4.0–11.0)*
Serum	
Urea *(mmol/l)*	4.3 *(2.5–6.7)*
Sodium *(mmol/l)*	136 *(134–145)*
Potassium *(mmol/l)*	3.7 *(3.5–5.0)*
Chloride *(mmol/l)*	101 *(95–105)*
Liver function tests	
Serum albumin *(g/l)*	32 *(35–50)*
Alkaline phosphatase *(IU/l)*	840 *(30–300)*
Alanine transaminase *(IU/ml)*	96 *(5–35)*
Aspartate transaminase *(IU/ml)*	148 *(5–35)*
Serum bilirubin *(µmol/l)*	29 *(3–17)*
Serology	
Hepatitis A	Negative
Hepatitis B	Negative
Hepatitis C	Negative
Clotting studies	
Prothrombin time *(secs)*	17.4 *(10–14)*
Activated partial thromboplastin time *(secs)*	54.0 *(35–50)*

Fig. 40.1 Results of investigations.

■ CASE 40 pp. 332–333

ANSWERS

1 What is the autoantigen in PBC?

The standard test for autoantibodies is indirect immunofluorescence which demonstrates AMA. The diagnosis of the disease is based on the finding of autoantibody but also a raised serum IgM. The AMA may be of the IgA or IgM class, and the titre may increase as the disease progresses. AMA is found in more than 95% of patients with PBC. AMA is found in other diseases such as cryptogenic cirrhosis (50% of cases) and chronic active hepatitis (40%), and in occasional cases of biliary obstruction.

The antigen to which the antibody is directed is located in the inner membrane of the mitochondria, although there are now other antigens described in the inner membrane which are not specific for PBC. The M2 antigen is specific for PBC and is a component of the 2-oxo acid dehydrogenase complex.

Other mitochondrial epitopes recognised by autoantibodies, all from the inner membrane, are the M1 cardiolipin seen in secondary syphilis and M7, seen in various cardiomyopathies.

2 What is thought to be the mechanism of damage to the liver?

Patients also have a wide variety of other autoantibodies including ANA and others directed against cytoskeleton, bile canaliculi and liver membrane. There is also evidence of increased synthesis and catabolism of C1q and C3, suggesting complement activation by antigen–antibody complexes. In spite of all these findings, no direct pathogenetic role has been identified for the AMA.

The antigens with which the AMA reacts do not seem to be specifically related to the liver, nor are they expressed on the bile canaliculi. More relevant are the antigens associated with the biliary tract. Two have been identified, one associated with the bile canalicular domain of the hepatocellular plasma membrane and the other with the surface of the bile duct epithelial cells. Cell mediated reactions have been shown with these two antigens which have also been identified in circulating immune complexes from patients with PBC.

The canalicular antigen cross-reacts with antigens in the kidney, pancreas and salivary ductules, which might explain some of the widespread clinical problems also seen in these patients. It is interesting that antibodies against group A streptococci cross-react with antigens in the biliary tract, kidney and salivary gland. This must raise a question as to whether PBC is a primary autoimmune disease or is an example of molecular mimicry.

3 What are the associated syndromes in patients with PBC?

Primary biliary cirrhosis occurs predominantly in women (9:1) and is characterised by slowly progressive obliteration of the intrahepatic bile ducts, which show epithelial cell damage with a surrounding lymphocyte infiltration. In the later stages granulomata can be seen with cirrhosis and piecemeal necrosis of the liver with fibrosis and also regeneration of the hepatocyte.

This can lead to jaundice with all the clinical sequelae associated with retained bile products. The diarrhoea is associated with poor fat absorption due to low levels of bile acids in the gut. This can then produce reduced absorption of fat soluble vitamins (A, D, E and K) with osteoporosis and osteomalacia. The mechanism of the bone abnormalities is not completely understood.

PBC can be described as a multisystem disease because of its association with the sicca syndrome and Sjögren's syndrome as well as abnormalities of the pancreas, thyroid, salivary and lacrimal glands. There are also features of the CREST syndrome (Calcinosis, Raynaud's phenomenon, Oesophageal dysmotility, Sclerodactyly, and Telangiectasia). There are also clinical associations with thyroiditis and rheumatoid arthritis. Clustering of cases is sometimes seen which indicates an environmental cause, perhaps a virus or bacteria as the aetiological agent.

It is possible to explain the association with the sicca syndrome by virtue of the cross-reaction of the canalicular antigen in the liver with that of the salivary glands. If this is the case, then damage to the secretory tubules would produce many of the clinical characteristics seen in both diseases (*Fig. 40.2*).

4 What treatment can be given to patients with PBC?

The diagnosis of PBC is often made on the basis of autoantibody tests when the patient has no symptoms at all. In these circumstances the patient needs no treatment. The onset of symptoms such as jaundice is a bad prognostic sign as the median survival at this stage is only 50% at 10 years.

Although there is no proven treatment for PBC, many immunosuppressive compounds have been tried. Azathioprine and D-penicillamine are ineffective. Cyclosporin A does slow the progression of the disease to some extent, but it causes renal damage and hypertension, thus limiting its value. Colchicine, acting also as an 'immunosuppressive' drug, is safe and does prolong survival compared with placebo. Methotrexate may be even more effective and has produced remissions in some patients before obvious cirrhosis is diagnosed. However, it is more toxic and some patients do develop an interstitial pneumonia which is reversible.

Sjögren's syndrome	Autoimmune thyroid disease
Sicca syndrome	SLE
Scleroderma	CREST syndrome
Rheumatoid arthritis	Mixed connective tissue disease
Dermatomyositis	Fibrosing alveolitis
	Renal tubular acidosis

Fig. 40.2 Syndromes associated with primary biliary cirrhosis.

CASE 41

Thirty-five-year-old Mrs Mozel was seen by a rheumatologist with increasing pain and stiffness in her fingers and wrists. Prior to her last pregnancy 2 years earlier she had experienced similar symptoms but they had receded following conception. Since the birth of the child, she had found it progressively more awkward to carry out a variety of tasks requiring fine finger co-ordination, including knitting, her favourite pastime. The symptoms were worse in the morning, although her hands felt clumsy throughout the day. Resting the hands seemed to worsen the degree of stiffness. Recently, she had also noticed a tingling sensation in the thumb and first two fingers of both hands which was worse at night.

She did not have any trouble with her other joints and had no visual disturbances or skin rashes. There was no history of rheumatic fever and she was otherwise well. Her mother had rheumatoid arthritis but her father was fit and well.

On examination Mrs Mozel was clinically anaemic but had no jaundice, oedema or lymphadenopathy, and was afebrile. She had bilateral and symmetrical tender swellings of her wrist and proximal interphalangeal and metacarpophalangeal joints, the latter being most marked. Ulnar deviation of the fingers was also present and she was unable to clench either hand to make a fist. There was no evidence of muscle wasting in the hands or arms. An examination of the elbow, shoulder, hip, knee and ankle joints did not show any swelling or tenderness, and there was a normal range of movement in each. The spine was similarly unaffected. Respiratory and cardiovascular examinations were unremarkable. Power in the intrinsic muscles of the hands was 4+ and sensation was normal to all modalities. An abdominal examination did not reveal any splenomegaly. The results of investigations are shown in *Figure 41.1*.

A diagnosis of early rheumatoid arthritis was made and Mrs Mozel was prescribed daily oral aspirin. This initially provided some relief of her symptoms, but also caused gastric irritation. She returned to her doctor 3 months later with worsening symptoms in her hands, and involvement of both her knees. On examination her metacarpophalangeal joints were swollen and very tender. Effusions were present in both her knees. Indomethacin was prescribed to control the effusions and the aspirin was discontinued.

Nine months after her first visit, Mrs Mozel developed bilateral subcutaneous nodules on the external surgaces of her forearms. These were 1 cm in diameter, firm, mobile, and non-tender. The tingling sensation in her hands she had described at her first visit had progressed to shooting pains alternating with numbness. The power in her thumb muscles was reduced and wasting was evident. Palmar erythema was noted bilaterally. The results of further investigations are shown in *Figure 41.2*.

A diagnosis of progressive rheumatoid arthritis with bilateral carpal tunnel syndrome was made. Mrs Mozel's dosage of indomethacin was increased and she was referred for physiotherapy.

QUESTIONS

1 How can rheumatoid arthritis be defined?
2 What genetic associations exist with rheumatoid arthritis?
3 What joint pathology is found in rheumatoid arthritis?
4 What is the immunopathogenesis of the disease?
5 What is rheumatoid factor?

Investigation	Result (normal range)
Haemoglobin (g/dl)	10.1 (11.5–16.0)
Platelet count (x 10⁹/l)	245 (150–400)
White cell count (x 10⁹/l)	12.5 (4.0–11.0)
Neutrophils (x 10⁹/l)	8.2 (2.0–7.5)
Total lymphocytes (x 10⁹/l)	2.1 (1.6–3.5)
Serum immunoglobulins	Normal
Serum albumin (g/l)	32 (35–50)
ESR	41 mm/hr
C reactive protein (mg/l)	25 (<5)
IgM rheumatoid factor	Positive
ANA	Negative
Antibodies to extractable nuclear antigens (ENA)	Negative
dsDNA binding activity	15%
Serum complement	
C3 (g/l)	1.02 (0.75–1.65)
C4 (g/l)	0.30 (0.20–0.65)
X-ray of hands	Osteopaenia of metacarpals and phalanges

Fig. 41.1 Results of investigations.

Investigation	Result (normal range)
Haemoglobin (g/dl)	10.4 (11.5–16.0)
White cell count (x 10⁹/l)	9.3 (4.0–11.0)
ESR	72 mm/hr
C reactive protein (mg/l)	68 (<5)
IgM rheumatoid factor	Positive
ANA	Negative
ENA	Negative
dsDNA binding activity	15%
Serum	
C3 (g/l)	0.98 (0.75–1.65)
C4 (g/l)	0.35 (0.20–0.65)
X-ray of hands	Erosions at the distal radii and metacarpophalangeal joints

Fig. 41.2 Results of further investigations.

■ CASE 41

pp. 329, 367–369

ANSWERS

1 How can rheumatoid arthritis be defined?

The term 'rheumatism' is derived from a Greek word meaning a stream or flow. It was first used in medieval times to describe pain caused by a deranged flow of one of the cardinal 'humours'. The name 'rheumatoid arthritis' (RA) was proposed by Garrod in 1859. The condition can be defined as a chronic, symmetrical, inflammatory polyarthritis of unknown cause involving the diathrodial joints and exhibiting, in a proportion of patients, extra-articular features. Estimates of the prevalence of the disease vary worldwide from 0.3% in Japan to 5.0% in Germany, with the UK figure at approximately 1%. There is a 3:1 female:male ratio in cases of RA (c.f. systemic lupus erythematosus 9:1 and Hashimoto's thyroiditis 25:1). Oestrogens may play a role in the pathogenesis of RA. It is known for example that pregnancy produces a protective or ameliorating effect, experienced by more than 75% of pregnant patients, usually in the third trimester.

2 What genetic associations exist with rheumatoid arthritis?

RA is an autoimmune disease associated with the HLA-DR4 and DR1 haplotypes. Detailed analysis of the molecular structure of the MHC II glycoprotein has revealed that susceptibility is, at least in part, governed by a five amino acid sequence found at positions 70–74 of the amino terminal domain of the HLA-DRβ chain. This sequence has been identified as glutamine-leucine-arginine-alanine-alanine, or glutamine-arginine-arginine-alanine-alanine. Two of the five subtypes of HLA-DR4, Dw4 and Dw14, possess these sequences as does the DR1 haplotype. Conversely, Dw10, which has different amino acids at positions 70 and 71, has no associated risk with RA. Some haplotypes, namely DR2, DR2 and DR3, and DR3 and DR7, exhibit a decreased risk of developing RA.

3 What joint pathology is found in rheumatoid arthritis?

In a RA joint, the synovium is turned from a relatively acellular structure into a proliferative and hypervascular lesion. It becomes infiltrated by immune cells and forms an invasive pannus which consists of a varied mixture of macrophages, mast cells, fibroblasts and cells with long processes. The junction between the invasive pannus and the joint cartilage is a focus for enzymatic degradation. Many of the cell types present appear to have a role in the destruction of cartilage found in RA.

In addition to the pannus there is lymphoid tissue organised around the synovial blood vessels. Lymphocytes are found peripheral to the vessels where they are surrounded by a transitional zone of macrophages, lymphocytes and differentiating B cells. The lymphocytes found near the blood vessels are largely CD4$^+$, whilst those in the transitional zone are a mixture of CD4$^+$ and CD8$^+$. There is contact between CD4$^+$ cells, B cells and HLA-DR$^+$ cells which resemble interdigitating cells and have antigen presenting function. This evidence points to a CD4$^+$ cell mediated process of clonal expansion within the synovium.

The synovial fluid of RA patients contains large numbers of polymorphonuclear leucocytes (PMNs) (up to 10^5/ml). Activation of the PMNs occurs following phagocytosis, particularly of IgG bound material, with subsequent release of oxygen radicals, arachidonic acid metabolites and IL-1.

4 What is the immunopathogenesis of the disease?

The specificity of the T-cell response in RA is unknown. The antigen may be a self-antigen, a modified self-antigen, a foreign antigen or a superantigen. A high proportion (70–90%) of RA patients have antibodies to a protein from the Epstein–Barr virus (EBV). These antibodies, named rheumatoid arthritis precipitin (RAP), cross react with a protein found in RA patients called rheumatoid arthritis nuclear antigen (RANA). RA patients also have elevated frequencies of EBV infected B cells compared with normal subjects. Furthermore, Gp110, a surface glycoprotein from EBV, possesses cross-reactive epitopes with the MHC II β-chain of HLA-Dw4, -Dw14 and -DR1. These amino acids are identical to the HLA sequences which confer susceptibility to RA. Infection with EBV in a genetically susceptible host could in theory trigger a clonal T-cell expansion directed against self-MHC II antigens.

Other candidate antigens include members of the heat shock protein (HSP) family. Certain lineages of $\gamma\delta$ T cells, which recognise HSP, have been isolated from RA patients. Recent data suggest a shared amino acid sequence between DR4, type XI collagen and *Proteus mirabilis*. This could be a further example of molecular mimicry producing disease.

5 What is rheumatoid factor?

Rheumatoid factors (RF) are autoantibodies that are able to bind IgG. RF exists in all five classes of immunoglobulin although the best characterised are IgG and IgM RF. Most RF bind to the Fc portion of the antibody, commonly at the CH2 and CH3 domains, although some react with the Fab regions. Around 70% of RA patients are RF seropositive. This group tends to develop a more aggressive disease.

Recent work suggests that the self-association found with IgG RF may be due to a deficiency in galactose residues bound via N-acetylglucosamine (GlcNAc) and mannose to a N-glycosylation site on the CH2 domain of the Fc region. It has been suggested that the absence of these sugar residues creates a galactose 'pocket' in the Fc region of the IgG RF enhancing self-association. Studies suggest that the prevalence of Gal(0) IgG, as it has been named, is increased in RA. Furthermore, it appears to be a marker of disease activity with reduced levels associated with, for example, the remission of RA found during pregnancy.

■ CASE 42

Mr Bell, a 50-year-old engineer, was seen by his GP with a 2-year history of painful joints. He had first noticed pain in his right foot, particularly at the metatarsophalangeal joint. Six months before visiting his doctor, he had developed intermittent sharp pain in his left shoulder and both elbows, which was worse in the morning and was aggravated by movement. His busy work schedule had prevented him seeking advice, but the rapid onset of pain and swelling of his finger, wrist, elbow, shoulder and knee joints had brought him to the attention of a rheumatologist. He also complained of lumbar and thoracic back pain, lethargy, malaise, fevers and a sore throat. All the symptoms had started while he was renovating his bathroom. He had no history of a rash, urethral discharge or conjunctivitis. There was no previous history of bruising or bleeding tendency.

Mr Bell was normally fit and well, and had no obvious HIV risk factors. He did not have a history of recurrent infections. Past medical history included a course of steroid treatment prescribed by a haematologist for a 'low white cell count'. As far as Mr Bell was concerned the matter had been resolved. He was an ex-smoker and moderate drinker. There was a suggestion that his mother, now very elderly, had suffered from rheumatoid arthritis in her middle age.

On examination, Mr Bell appeared well, but a little overweight. There was no evidence of a rash or lymphadenopathy. There was a mild pyrexia of 37.5°C. He had bilateral olecranon bursae and early subcutaneous nodule formation. A degree of subluxation was noted at the metatarsophalangeal joints of the right foot with some tender swelling of the joints of his hands,

elbows, shoulders and knees. Cardiovascular, respiratory and abdominal examinations were all unremarkable. Results of investigations are shown in *Figure 42.1*.

A diagnosis of Felty's syndrome was made and Mr Bell was treated with a course of prednisolone for his neutropaenia and Myocrisin (gold) injections for his arthritis. His full blood counts were watched judiciously throughout treatment, as gold can provoke neutropaenia. His joint symptoms resolved within 3 months, and his neutrophil count returned to normal. He did not have any significant infectious episodes during treatment. He was maintained on monthly gold injections.

Two years later, Mr Bell had a further episode of neutropaenia, with counts persistently below $0.3 \times 10^9/1$. Pulses of intravenous methylprednisolone were required to increase his count. Further investigations were carried out at this time (*Fig. 42.2*).

There was an absence of late segmented neutrophils compatible with peripheral sequestration found in Felty's syndrome.

A diagnosis of large granular lymphocyte (LGL) syndrome was made, and the possibility was also raised of idiopathic CD4 lymphopaenia.

QUESTIONS

1 What is Felty's syndrome and does it have a genetic basis?
2 What is the cause of the neutropaenia in Felty's syndrome?
3 What is the LGL syndrome?
4 What is known of idiopathic CD4 lymphopaenia?

Investigation	Result *(normal range)*
Haemoglobin *(g/dl)*	15.7 *(11.5–16.0)*
White cell count *(x 10⁹/l)*	2.5 *(4.0–11.0)*
Neutrophil count *(x 10⁹/l)*	0.4 *(2.0–7.5)*
Lymphocyte count *(x 10⁹/l)*	1.2 *(1.6–3.5)*
Platelet count *(x 10⁹/l)*	248 *(150–400)*
ESR *(mm/hr)*	130 *(<20)*
C reactive protein *(mg/l)*	145 *(<5)*
Rheumatoid slide latex	Positive 1.160
Autoantibodies	
ANA	Positive 1/40
DNA binding	Positive 501
Anti-dsDNA	Positive
Anti-neutrophil antibodies	Positive, surface bound IgG
Other	All negative
Radiographs of feet	Bilateral halux valgus, no evidence of erosions
Ultrasound of liver and spleen	Normal liver, homogenously enlarged spleen

Fig. 42.1 Results of investigations.

Investigation	Result *(normal range)*
Haemoglobin *(g/dl)*	15.7 *(11.5–16.0)*
White cell count *(x 10⁹/l)*	2.8 *(4.0–11.0)*
Neutrophil count *(x 10⁹/l)*	1.2 *(2.0–7.5)*
Lymphocyte count *(x 10⁹/l)*	1.2 *(1.6–3.5)*
Platelet count *(x 10⁹/l)*	150 *(150–400)*
CD3⁺	1170
CD3⁺	91% *(60–85)*
CD19⁺	48
CD19⁺	4% *(7–23)*
CD4⁺	188
CD4⁺	15% *(29–59)*
CD8⁺	852
CD8⁺	66% *(19–48)*
CD4/CD8 ratio	0.2 *(0.6–2.8)*
% of CD16⁺ lymphocytes	60
Bone marrow aspirate	Absence of late segmented neutrophils compatible with peripheral sequestration found in Felty's syndrome

Fig. 42.2 Results of further investigations.

■ CASE 42

Chapter 28

ANSWERS

1 What is Felty's syndrome and does it have a genetic basis?

Felty's syndrome (FS) is a triad of rheumatoid arthritis (RA), neutropaenia and splenomegaly initially characterised by A R Felty in 1924. Approximately 1–3% of patients with RA have Felty's syndrome. The splenomegaly is variable both in timing and extent, and is not found in some subjects. Such patients share the same clinical and immunological features of classical FS, thus the splenomegaly can no longer be considered an obligatory part of the syndrome. More than 90% of patients are HLA-DR4 positive, compared with 70% of RA patients and 30% of the general population. The DW4, DW14 (DRB1*0401, DRB1*0404/8) combination is particularly common in FS. These data strongly implicate the role of an antigen-dependent CD4+ T-cell mediated step in the pathogenesis of FS.

The neutropaenia of FS may be mild to severe, fluctuating, or resolve completely in some patients. In general the degree of neutropaenia correlates withthe incidence of infection. An absolute neutrophil count of less than 1000 significantly increases the risk of infection, which is usually bacterial and may be fatal. Additional factors contributing to the immunodeficiency may include CD4+ lymphopaenia reported in some patients, although the degree of lymphopaenia is not usually as profound as the 188/µl in Mr Bell's case. Hypocomplementaemia, immune complexes and granulocyte dysfunction are all thought to contribute to decreased immune responsiveness. Thrombocytopaenia and/or anaemia are variable features of FS.

2 What is the cause of the neutropaenia in Felty's syndrome?

The cause of neutropaenia varies between subjects. In some, arrested development of neutrophils in the bone marrow is the predominant mechanism. This may occur by two methods:

- The activity of suppressor cells, possibly CD4+.
- Decreased granulopoietin production.
  Other causes of the neutropaenia appear to include:
- Circulating immune complexes enhancing complement fixation.
- Neutrophil sequestration in the spleen. Anti-neutrophil antibodies implicated in sequestration are directed against both cell-surface antigens and, more prominently, to cytoplasmic antigens, with 77% of patients in one series aspecific ANCA positive.

3 What is the LGL syndrome?

The large granular lymphocyte syndrome (LGL) is characterised by the expansion of LGLs in peripheral blood. Most, but not all, LGLs possess 'natural killer' (NK) activity. These cells do not possess a T-cell receptor, although most are CD16 (FcγRIII) positive. Killing therefore occurs in non-major histo-compatibility complex restricted fashion, and represents a first line of defence to infection with a peak response 3 days after inoculation.

The T cell LGL syndrome is far the most common variety, and is often clonal. Approximately 30% of patients with the LGL syndrome have RA, with many also having neutropenia and splenomegaly. Conversely, 19–35% of patients with FS have clonal LGL expansion. The neutropaenia is closely associated with clonality of the LGLs. There is considerable controversy as to whether this syndrome is 'pre-malignant'.

4 What is known of idiopathic CD4 lymphopaenia?

Idiopathic CD4 lymphopaenia is defined as the presence of a CD4 count less than 300 cells/mm³ or less than 20% of the total T-cell count, on more than one occasion. Furthermore, there must be no evidence of infection on HIV testing, and no defined immunodeficiency or therapy associated with depressed levels of CD4+ T cells. The clinical features of these patients differ from those with HIV infection in that.

- There is no evidence of HIV-1, HIV-2; HTLV-1, HTLV-2 either by antibody screening or polymerase chain reaction.
- The condition is extremely rare.
- The condition is probably not new (unlike the comparatively recent onset of HIV).
- Many patients do not have a deteriorating clinical course but remain stable.
- A proportion of patients have spontaneous recovery of their CD4 count.
- The age range is wide (17–78 years in one series).
- Immunoglobulin levels are usually normal or low in contrast to the hypergammaglobulinaemia of HIV infection.
- Low CD8 counts are also found in a proportion (25% in one study).

In conclusion, the following can be said:

- Idiopathic CD4 T-lymphocytopaenia is probably a misnomer; some cases probably have an underlying non-HIV infectious cause.
- In a proportion of cases the result may reflect inaccurate laboratory methods.
- The CD4 count does not correlate with the type of complication seen.

CASE 43

Twenty-five-year-old Miss Heller had not felt well for some time but put all her symptoms down to a change of job which was much more stressful. She had felt tired and, unusually for her, had lost her appetite. She had then developed increasing abdominal pain, aching joints and a skin rash.

She was admitted to hospital with a history of fatigue and, in addition, amenorrhoea. She had no history of intravenous drug misuse and no family history of malignancy or liver disease. She was asked if she had ever had hepatitis or jaundice and she assured the doctors that this had never been the case. Medical history of note was hypothyroidism diagnosed 5 years earlier for which she was receiving thyroxine supplements. She was not on any other medication.

On examination, Miss Heller had palmar erythema, numerous spider naevi and an enlarged liver and spleen, and was clearly jaundiced. No Kayser–Fleisher rings were seen. The results of investigations are shown in *Figure 43.1*.

A diagnosis of autoimmune chronic active hepatitis (CAH) was made and Miss Heller was started on corticosteroid and vitamin K therapy. Within a fortnight her liver function test results had returned to normal and her symptoms had improved. She was discharged on a maintenance dosage of corticosteroids and was reviewed regularly.

QUESTIONS

1 What are the possible causes of CAH?
2 What autoantibodies are found in CAH?
3 What are the immunological mechanisms of damage?

Investigation	Result (normal range)
Haemoglobin (g/dl)	9.8 (11.5–16.0)
White cell count (x 10⁹/l)	6.9 (4.0–11.0)
Liver function tests	
Aspartate aminotransferase (IU/ml)	86 (5–35)
Alanine aminotransferase (IU/ml)	91 (5–35)
Alkaline phosphatase (IU/l)	523 (30–300)
Serum albumin (g/l)	31 (35–50)
Clotting studies	
Prothrombin time (secs)	19.1 (10–14)
Activated partial thromboplastin time (secs)	53.3 (35–45)
Serology	
Hepatitis A	Negative
Hepatitis B	Negative
Hepatitis C	Negative
Serum immunoglobulins	
IgG (g/l)	19.3 (5.4–16.1)
IgM (g/l)	1.2 (0.5–1.9)
IgA (g/l)	1.4 (0.8–2.8)
Autoantibodies	
ANA	Positive
Anti-dsDNA	Positive
Anti-smooth muscle	Positive
Liver biopsy	Piecemeal necrosis and evidence of cirrhosis. T cells and plasma cells present

Fig. 43.1 Results of investigations.

■ CASE 43   pp. 367–369

ANSWERS

1 What are the possible causes of CAH?

There has been much discussion as to the exact diagnostic criteria for CAH. Initially, the finding of 'piecemeal necrosis' was considered diagnostic. This can be defined as ballooning degeneration and necrosis of hepatocytes along the edge of portal tracts, fibrous septa or zones of necrosis. However, this is not limited to CAH but can also be found in other liver diseases such as acute viral hepatitis, Wilson's disease, primary biliary cirrhosis and alcoholic hepatitis.

Other conditions such as chronic hepatitis associated with HBsAg, drugs and α1-antitrypsin deficiency can also produce a similar picture.

Following acute hepatitis B, approximately 1 in 10 patients become chronic carriers – most of them being asymptomatic. Some however do progress to chronic hepatitis, giving a histological presentation similar to that seen in CAH. With hepatitis C, almost two-thirds of the patients who develop post-transfusion hepatitis develop chronic liver disease. These patients frequently progress to CAH.

The classic form of CAH, which has been termed lupoid chronic hepatitis, has no obvious cause but 20% of patients do have ANAs. These patients are mainly women and the onset of the disease can often be traced back to an acute viral illness.

2 What autoantibodies are found in CAH?

It is now possible to subdivide CAH into two main categories, as are shown in Appendix 5). Classical autoimmune CAH (AI-CAH), associated with ANA and anti-smooth muscle antibody (SMA), is now designated Type 1. Type 2 is found in those patients where there is the presence of liver/kidney/microsomal antibody (LKM). There is also a group of patients who are seronegative, but who show the same histopathology of the liver.

There are various patterns of ANA which can give further diagnostic help. Homogeneous staining of the nucleus is seen in SLE, speckled in the extractable nuclear antigen (ENA) syndromes, nucleolar in scleroderma, peripheral in various syndromes, and centromere staining in the CREST syndrome. The ANA in AI-CAH is homogeneous and similar to that seen in SLE. There is also some staining against dsDNA but to different epitopes to that seen in SLE.

The SMA had previously been thought to be specific for smooth muscle protein and in particular the smooth muscle protein F-actin. It is now clear that SMA also occurs in other diseases. In addition, although the majority of CAH patients have SMA, only half show anti-actin specificity.

There are a number of LKM autoantibodies, most reacting with cytochrome P450 enzymes. Of these, LKM1 seems to predict Type 2 AI-CAH. This antibody reacts with cytochrome P450 IID6 which was formerly known as P450db1. In a study of patients with Type 2 AI-CAH who showed high titres of LKM1, the majority were shown to have antibodies to hepatitis C and 70% were viraemic, as shown by the polymerase chain reaction-based assay for serum hepatitis C virus RNA. It would seem likely that hepatitis C virus plays a major role in the aetiology of Type 2 AI-CAH.

A number of other autoantibodies are seen in CAH, including anti-thyroid, reticulin, and gastric parietal cell as well as rheumatoid factor.

3 What are the immunological mechanisms of damage?

Autoantibodies are sometimes a significant marker of autoimmune disease but may not be directly pathogenetic. This is the case with the autoantibodies described so far.

Two autoantibodies may be more relevant. One is directed against a liver-specific membrane lipoprotein (LSP) which in reality is a crude fraction of normal liver containing hepatocellular membranes with a number of antigens. The other, the asialoglycoprotein receptor (ASGP-R), has been identified from this mixture. This is the receptor which binds glycoproteins and aids endocytosis of those bearing terminal galactose residues. Relevant to the disease, this receptor is specific to the liver and is expressed on cells in the periportal area of the liver. This happens to be the site of major damage in CAH.

The damage to the liver involves cell infiltration and tests of cellular immune function may be more relevant than an assay of autoantibodies. Using leucocyte migration inhibition as a measure of cell mediated immunity, patients with CAH react positively to LSP and ASGP-R. This is not seen in hepatitis B virus induced cases. In co-culture experiments, T cells from normal controls were able to block the response of patients' cells in the assay. It is possible that patients have a defect of suppression in controlling the autoreactive response to this antigen. T-cell cloning supports these observations in that cells from AI-CAH patients recognise ASGP-R, are CD4+ and provide *in vitro* help for production of ASGP-R autoantibodies.

It is likely that a virus is required to initiate the disease in a susceptible person, where the absence of adequate suppression allows the autoimmune process to proceed unchecked.

CASE 44

When Lucy went to her GP complaining of feeling tired, she was told that it was studying for her university entrance exams that was the cause. Her doctor did not bother to examine her at that time. She did well enough in her exams but did not feel able to take up the university place that was offered and asked to be deferred for 1 year. During the next few months, she lost her appetite and started to lose weight. She had occasional attacks of vomiting and diarrhoea, which she put down to food poisoning. Although she had no formal studying to do, she became increasingly tired and irritable.

She went back to her GP and explained all her symptoms which now included muscle weakness, sweats and some abdominal problems. He did examine her on this occasion and was surprised to find her blood pressure low at 90/60 mmHg, and noted that she did seem to have a good sun tan. When the doctor examined Lucy further he found pigmentation of her nail beds, areolae, gum margins and buccal mucosa. He enquired whether she had any previous infections with *Candida albicans*.

The family history was interesting; her mother had thyroid disease and a sister had been recently diagnosed as an insulin dependent diabetic. A number of investigations were ordered, the results of which are shown in *Figure 44.1*.

The plain X-ray of her abdomen was to exclude calcification in the adrenal area which might have suggested tuberculosis. There was also no evidence of malignancy that may be affecting the adrenal glands. The further series of tests that were made showed quite clearly that her adrenal function was poor and that cortisol production was not increased following the injection of adrenocorticotrophic hormone (ACTH).

With the tests of autoantibodies being positive, in conjunction with the family history, a diagnosis of autoimmune Addison's disease was made. Following treatment, Lucy felt very much better, regained her health quickly and resumed her university career.

QUESTIONS

1 What is the evidence for immune involvement in Addison's disease?
2 What are the major auto antigens in autoimmune Addison's disease?
3 What other endocrine diseases are associated with Addison's disease?
4 What used to be the major cause of Addison's disease?
5 How is Addison's disease treated?

Investigation	Result *(normal range)*
Haemoglobin *(g/dl)*	13.9 *(11.5–16.0)*
White cell count *(x 10⁹/l)*	9.3 *(4.0–11.0)*
Serum	
Sodium *(mmol/l)*	130 *(134–145)*
Potassium *(mmol/l)*	5.2 *(3.5–5.0)*
Chloride *(mmol/l)*	94 *(95–105)*
Urea *(mmol/l)*	8.1 *(2.5–6.7)*
Glucose *(mmol/l)*	2.3 *(>10)*
Serum cortisol at 9:00 am *(nmol/l)*	85 *(280–700)*
ACTH stimulation test	
Cortisol at 1 hr *(nmol/l)*	100 *(>500)*
Autoantibodies	
Anti-adrenal cortex cytoplasm	Positive
Abdominal X-ray	Normal
Abdominal ultrasound	Normal

Fig. 44.1 Results of investigations.

■ CASE 44   pp. 367–369

ANSWERS

1 What is the evidence for immune involvement in Addison's disease?

There are several strands of evidence pointing to immunological involvement in autoimmune Addison's disease. There is often a strong family history of autoimmune disease, which was the case in Lucy's family. The link with thyroid and autoimmune gastritis is not common but does occur. There is also a high incidence of other autoantibodies in these patients.

The histology of the adrenal gland in idiopathic Addison's disease shows marked lymphocytic infiltration characteristic of that seen in other autoimmune diseases. Cell mediated immunity can be shown by reacting the patient's lymphocytes to adrenal cortex tissue *in vitro* when activation occurs.

Lastly, immunisation of animals with adrenal tissue in complete Freund's adjuvant reproduces adrenalitis, with a histological picture similar to that seen in the human. Passive transfer of cells from an immunised to a control animal leads to the disease and adrenal failure in the recipient animal.

2 What are the major autoantigens in autoimmune Addison's disease?

The standard assay for autoantibodies is indirect immunofluorescence on the target tissue, in this case, the adrenal gland. Fluorescence is seen in the adrenal cortex with cells in the zona glomerulosa staining positive. Fractionation of the adrenal cortex shows antibody binding in the subcellular fractions enriched for microsomal enzymes. In a small number of patients with Addison's disease there is also gonadal failure. These patients have antibodies directed not only against the adrenal but also against extra-adrenal steroid producing organs.

Polyendocrine autoimmunity is defined as two or more endocrine autoimmune diseases in the same person. It can be classified into two main groups both of which can suffer from Addison's disease. These are summarised in *Figure 44.2*. Type 1 is associated with mucocutaneous *Candida* and has a higher frequency of antibodies against gonadal steroid producing cells. Type 2 is later in onset and lacks gonadal dysfunction.

	Type 1	Type 2
Onset	Early	Late
Antibody to adrenal gland	+	+
Antibody to gonad cells	+	–
HLA association	–	HLA DR3
Mucocutaneous *Candida*	+	–
Association with other autoimmune diseases	+	+
Gonads affected	+	–
Autoantigen	17α hydroxylase	21 hydroxylase
MW (kDa)	55	54

Fig. 44.2 Comparison of type I and II polyendocrinopathy.

The autoantigens have now been defined as enzymes associated with the steroid synthesis pathway. 17α hydroxylase is necessary for the production of cortisol, progesterone, oestrogen and testosterone. 21 Hydroxylase is required to produce corticosterone and aldosterone. These findings fit in with the biochemical abnormalities in the patients.

It is interesting that a number of other autoantigens are also enzymes; thyroid peroxidase in Hashimoto's disease; H^+K^+-ATPase in autoimmune gastritis; cytochrome P450-dbI in autoimmune hepatitis Type II; glutamate decarboxylase in Type I insulin dependent diabetes mellitus.

3 What other endocrine diseases are associated with Addison's disease?

Ovarian failure is seen in approximately 25% of cases of Addison's disease and this correlates with the presence of antibodies directed against steroid producing cells. These antibodies are generally detected by immunofluorescence or more recently by Western blot analysis. *Candida* endocrinopathy can be associated with a number of organ specific autoimmune diseases as in Schmidt's syndrome. This consists of hypoparathyroidism, mucocutaneous *Candida* and organ specific autoimmune disease. Patients can also suffer from vitiligo. This is seen in cases of Type 1 polyendocrinopathy, which has these features as well as gonadal failure. In Type 2 disease, adrenal failure is not usually associated with gonadal dysfunction but with Graves' disease, insulin dependent diabetes mellitus, coeliac disease and myasthenia gravis.

Type 2 polyendocrinopathy is much more common than Type 1 and is likely to be an autosomal dominant disorder. Separate components of the autoimmune disorder can present many years apart and long-term follow-up of these patients is important.

Both Type 1 and Type 2 are associated with vitiligo, alopecia and pernicious anaemia.

4 What used to be the major cause of Addison's disease?

When chronic infections were more common than now, the usual cause of Addison's disease was tuberculosis of the adrenal gland. This was the rationale for asking for an abdominal X-ray to see if there was any calcification in the adrenal area. In recent years, tuberculosis has become a rare cause of Addison's disease, but with its resurgence as a disease common in AIDS patients, and with the increase of the disease in inner city areas, it is likely that infectious causes for Addison's disease will again become more prominent.

5 How is Addison's disease treated?

Treatment is replacement of steroids and mineralocorticoids as indicated by the biochemical tests. Lucy had evidence of corticosteroid deficiency as shown by the low adrenal reserve in the ACTH stimulation tests as well as aldosterone deficiency as shown by her electrolyte balance. Replacement of each segment resulted in a return to good health.

CASE 45

When David was 16 years old he started to complain of pains in his joints and in his back. One of the areas that hurt was his lower back and he would often get out of bed in the early hours of the morning and try and get comfortable either by laying on the floor or by sitting in a chair. He was always stiff in the mornings and he would try and exercise to get himself supple so that he could start the day being more comfortable. He also had pains in his heels which were very disturbing and made it difficult to walk.

The pains continued for some months and he became tired and much less able to cope at school. He also developed pains in his knees. At one stage he had a red eye which was treated by his own doctor.

He eventually reached a specialist rheumatologist who found a number of abnormalities when he examined him. When he asked David to touch his toes there was limited flexion of the spine. He also found that David's spine was slightly bowed, his hips lacked mobility, and his knees and heels were painful. He had a mild iritis, and there was a macular rash on his trunk. The results of investigations are shown in *Figure 45.1*.

The finding of HLA B27 on tissue typing led to the diagnosis of ankylosing spondylitis.

Exercise and anti-inflammatory drugs relieved many, but not all, of the symptoms. David was then put on a low carbohydrate diet and within a few weeks he felt very much better. By the end of 2 months on the diet, his ESR and C reactive protein had returned to normal levels. Total IgA was increased and antibodies to *Klebsiella pneumoniae* were present in high titre. These returned to normal levels after more months on the diet. He remained well, keeping to his diet and taking non-steroidal anti-inflammatory drugs (NSAIDs) when necessary.

QUESTIONS

1 What percentage of patients with ankylosing spondylitis (AS) are HLA B27 positive?
2 What is the significance of antibodies to *Klebsiella pneumoniae*?
3 Could this disease be caused by molecular mimicry? If so, what experiments might you do to investigate this possibility?

Investigation	Result (normal range)
Haemoglobin (g/l)	10.1 (11.5–16.0)
White cell count (x 10⁹/l)	8.1 (4.0–11.0)
ESR	92 mm/hr
C reactive protein (mg/l)	32 (<5)
Immunoglobulins	
IgG (g/l)	8.4 (5.4–16.1)
IgM (g/l)	2.2 (0.5–1.9)
IgA (g/l)	6.4 (0.8–2.8)
Autoantibodies	
Rheumatoid factor	Negative
ANA	Negative
Chest X-ray	Normal
X-ray pelvis	Evidence of sacroiliitis
X-ray of spine	Early signs of ossification of the anterior tissues of the lumbar vertebrae
HLA typing	B27 positive

Fig. 45.1 Results of investigations.

■ **CASE 45**   pp. 367–369

ANSWERS

1 What percentage of patients with ankylosing spondylitis are HLA B27 positive?

Ankylosing spondylitis (AS) is one of the forms of spondyl-arthritis which affect mainly the spine, although other joints can be affected, such as the shoulder and pelvic girdle. The group of seronegative spondylarthropathies can be divided into four, namely: AS, reactive arthritis, the arthritis associated with inflammatory bowel disease (Crohn's disease and ulcerative colitis) and psoriatic arthritis. Unlike most forms of arthritis, it is more common in men, with onset in the late teens or early twenties, and is seronegative, i.e. the patients do not have autoantibodies or rheumatoid factor. Patients may also develop uveitis.

AS is the purest form of spondylarthritis, and 95% of the patients are HLA-B27 positive, in contrast with the low frequency (around 8%) of HLA B27 in the Caucasian population. This phenotype is useful for diagnosis, as AS is unlikely to be present in a patient who does not have B27. The relative risk for AS in B27 positive individuals is more than 300. It is difficult to estimate how many individuals who are B27 positive have AS and figures ranging from 1% to 20% are given.

It is clear that B27 is a susceptibility gene in human AS. Further evidence to support this is the use of a rat transgene which contains multiple copies of the B27 gene. These rats develop arthritis and a syndrome that is similar to AS.

2 What is the significance of antibodies to *Klebsiella pneumoniae*?

Since the description of the seronegative spondylarthropathies, it has been realised that many of them are strongly linked to HLA B27. Reactive arthritis following a gut infection shares many similarities with AS, raising the possibility that they might all be related to a gut infection in some way. Reiter's disease is associated with infection by *Yersinia enterocolitica* and this shares some similar surface epitopes with the arthritogenic *Shigella flexneri*.

Ebringer was the first to show that patients with AS had increased levels of *Klebsiella pneumoniae* in the stool and the disease activity was related to the microbial burden. None of the other cross-reacting micro-organisms was found in the stool of AS patients. Active inflammatory disease was associated with an increase in total serum IgA, supporting the idea that the organism was acting at a mucosal surface in the gut.

The specificity of antibodies to *K. pneumoniae* was then tested and it became clear-cut that IgA antibodies are present in high titres in AS patients but not in controls or in patients with rheumatoid arthritis.

It is relevant that AS patients do have gut problems, and two-thirds of them have subclinical inflammatory lesions of the bowel. There are a number of possible ways of reducing the *K. pneumoniae* population to see if the patient improves

symptomatically. A diet low in carbohydrate starves out the organisms and does produce clinical improvement in the patients. In addition, salazopyrine also reduces the load of organisms and again is associated with clinical improvement. This evidence supports the central role of *Klebsiella* in the inflammatory process in AS.

3 Could this disease be caused by molecular mimicry? If so, what experiments might you do to investigate this possibility?

A theory which suggests molecular mimicry implies that epitopes on an environmental agent such as a micro-organism, in this case *K. pneumoniae*, resemble a similar sequence in the HLA molecule, in this case HLA B27. There are a number of clinical situations where molecular mimicry exists, such as in rheumatic fever, where epitopes are shared between the streptococci and heart valve.

A more formal approach is to use antisera against both *K. pneumoniae* and B27 to see if there is any cross reaction. If monoclonal antibodies against HLA B27 are used to stain various bacteria, strong reactions are seen with *Klebsiella*, *Yersinia* and *Shigella*. The reverse experiment has also been done, namely, staining lymphoid cell lines with antibodies directed against *K. pneumoniae*. When this has been done, lines expressing B27 stain positively with the antibacterial antibody, although cells with surface HLA B7 also stained. This antigen cross reacts with B27.

What is the explanation for the site of the inflammation in AS? There is fibrosis and calcification along the vertebrae and also localisation of inflammatory foci at regions of ligament or tendon insertions into bone. Using monoclonal antibodies against *K. pneumoniae* and B27, there is extensive expression of structures reacting to both of the antisera. Particular staining was seen within synovial lining cells of the joints and in endothelial cells of blood vessels in tissues affected by the AS process. Unfortunately, these particular studies do not explain the localisation of the disease along the vertebral bodies.

However, if the main cross-reacting antigen from *K. pneumoniae* is in the gut wall, it may be that antibody would be found in high titres in the draining lymph nodes which are linked anatomically to the lumbar spine and sacroiliac joints. It is not unreasonable that these areas would bear the brunt of the ensuing inflammation.

Lastly, the structure that provides the cross-reacting epitope has been defined. Oldstone has identified a hexamer amino acid sequence, Gln-Thr-Asp-Arg-Glu-Asp, which is present in both HLA B27 and *K. pneumoniae* and in fact represents the epitope of the nitrogenase reductase enzyme. Patients with AS do have antibodies against this sequence.

This model of molecular mimicry can provide an explanation of AS, with the epitope now narrowed down to an area spanning only six amino acids.

Test	Age / Sex	Normal range	
Haemoglobin	Man	13.5–18.0 g/dl	
	Woman	11.5–16.0 g/dl	
	Cord	>16.0 g/dl	
MCV		78–96 fl	
MCH		27–32 pg	
MCHC		30–34 g/dl	
Serum iron		12–32 mmol/l	
TIBC		45–72 mmol/l	
Serum B12		150–900 ng/l	
Red cell folate		160–640 ng/l	
Prothrombin time		10–14 secs	
Activated partial thromboplastin time		35–45 secs	
White cell count	<12 mths	6.4–11.0 x 10⁹/l	
	1–6 yrs	6.8–10.0 x 10⁹/l	
	>6 yrs	4.0–11.0 x 10⁹/l	
Neutrophils		2.0–7.5 x 10⁹/l	40–75% WCC
Eosinophils		0.4–0.44 x 10⁹/l	1–6% WCC
Basophils		0.01–0.10 x 10⁹/l	0–1% WCC
Monocytes		0.2–0.8 x 10⁹/l	1–10% WCC
Total lymphocytes	<12 mths	2.7–5.4 x 10⁹/l	
	1–17 yrs	2.0–4.1 x 10⁹/l	20–45% WCC
	>17 yrs	1.6–3.5 x 10⁹/l	
T lymphocytes	1–6 yrs	2.7–5.3 x 10⁹/l	
	7–17 yrs	2.0–2.7 x 10⁹/l	
	>17 yrs	1.6–2.4 x 10⁹/l	
CD4⁺	<12 mths	1.7–2.8 x 10⁹/l	
	1–6 yrs	1.0–1.8 x 10⁹/l	
	>6 yrs	0.7–1.1 x 10⁹/l	
CD8⁺	0–6 yrs	0.8–1.5 x 10⁹/l	
	>6 yrs	0.5–0.9 x 10⁹/l	
B lymphocytes	0–6 yrs	0.6–1.4 x 10⁹/l	
	>6 yrs	0.2–0.5 x 10⁹/l	
Platelets		150–400 x 10⁹/l	

Appendix 1a Normal ranges of haematology and blood chemistry measurements.

Test	Normal range
Blood gases	
PaO₂	>10.6 kPa
PaCO₂	4.7–6.0 kPa
pH	7.35–7.45
Serum electrolytes	
Sodium	134–145 mmol/l
Potassium	3.5–5.0 mmol/l
Chloride	95–105 mmol/l
Calcium (total)	2.12–2.65 mmol/l
Phosphate	0.8–1.45 mmol/l
Urea	2.5–6.7 mmol/l
Creatinine	70–150 µmol/l
Liver function tests	
Alkaline phosphatase	30–300 IU/l
Aspartate transaminase	5–35 IU/ml
Alanine transaminase	5–35 IU/ml
Total serum bilirubin	3–17 µmol/l
Serum albumin	35–50 g/l
Total serum protein	60–80 g/l
Fasting blood glucose	4.0–6.7 mmol/l
Random blood glucose	<10.0 mmol/l
CSF	
Glucose	>60% of blood glucose
Protein	0.15–0.45 g/l
Cells	0–5 lymphocytes/mm³
Serum parathyroid hormone	0.1–0.73 µg/l
Serum cortisol at 9.00am	280–700 nmol/l
Serum cortisol 1 hr after ACTH	>500 nmol/l
Serum angiotensin converting enzyme	male 22–82 u/l / female 25–69 u/l
Serum T3	1.2–3.0 nmol/l
Serum free T4	9–22 pmol/l
TSH	0.5–5.7 mU/l
Faecal fat	<6g/24 hr

Appendix 1b Normal ranges of chemical pathology.

Age	IgE IU/ml	IgM g/l	IgA g/l	IgG g/l	IgG1 g/l	IgG2 g/l	IgG3 g/l	IgG4 g/l
<6 months	0.3–20	0.02–2.10	0.1–0.5	2.4–8.8	1.5–6.8	0.5–5.8	0.2–1.2	0.15–0.95
<2 years	3–22	0.4–2.2	0.15–1.3	3.0–15.8	1.5–9.8	0.3–3.9	0.1–0.8	0.05–0.65
2–4 years	3–150	0.5–2.0	0.3–2.0	3.7–16.1	4.3–12.7	0.3–4.4	0.1–1.0	0.10–0.84
4–6 years	3–150	0.5–2.0	0.4–2.0	4.9–16.1	5.6–11.3	0.4–4.0	0.3–0.8	0.14–0.95
6–12 years	3–150	0.5–1.8	0.5–2.5	5.4–16.1	6.2–11.5	0.5–4.8	0.3–1.0	0.20–0.93
>12 years	3–150	0.5–1.9	0.8–2.8	5.4–16.1	4.8–9.5	1.7–6.9	0.3–0.8	0.23–1.11

Appendix 2a Normal ranges of immunoglobulin classes and IgG subclasses.

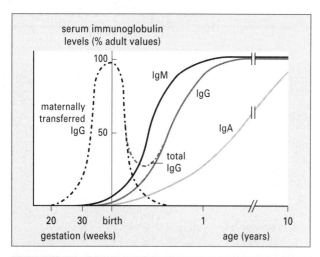

Appendix 2b Serum immunoglobulin and IgG subclasses vary with age. In the newborn child, the bulk of the circulating IgG is from the mother until the age of 3 months. The level of IgA reaches adult proportions by the age of 10 years.

Test	Normal range
Complement:	
C1q	100–250 mg/l
C2	10–30 mg/l
C3	0.75–1.65 g/l
C4	0.20–0.65 g/l
C1INH	0.15–0.35 g/l
ESR	Male: age divided by 2
	Female: age + 10 divided by 2
C reactive protein	<5 mg/l
Serum β_2 microglobulin	1.2–2.4 mg/l
Anti-D antibodies	<1.0 IU/ml – no action required
	>5.0 IU/ml rising rapidly – action required
	>10.0 IU/ml – action required

Appendix 3 Normal values: Complement components and anti-D antibodies. Complement levels will vary if there is a significant inflammatory disease. As they can also be classed as acute phase proteins, the blood levels may be raised. C1 inhibitor levels are low in hereditary angioedema (HAE). However, the antigenic level may be normal but the C1 may be fractional. The function should be measured if there is clinical doubt as to the diagnosis of HAE.

Vaccine	Type	Route	Age	Notes
Diphtheria	Toxoid	IM	2,3 & 4 months	
Tetanus	Toxoid	IM	2,3 & 4 months	
Pertussis	Killed organism	IM	2,3 & 4 months	
HiB	Polysaccharides	IM	2,3 & 4 months	
Polio, Sabin	Live attenuated	PO	2,3 & 4 months	
Measles	Live attenuated	IM	12–18 months	Given later if necessary
Mumps	Live attenuated	IM	12–18 months	Given later if necessary
Rubella	Live attenuated	IM	12–18 months	Given later if necessary
Diphtheria	Toxoid	IM	School entry	Booster
Tetanus	Toxoid	IM	School entry	Booster
Polio, Sabin	Live attenuated	PO	School entry	Booster
Rubella	Live attenuated	ID	10–14 years	Girls only
BCG (TB)	Live attenuated	ID	10–14 years	After negative Heaf test
Tetanus	Toxoid	IM	15–18 years	Booster
Polio, Sabin	Live attenuated	PO	15–18 years	Booster

Appendix 4 Vaccination schedules. MMR vaccine has been commonly contraindicated in children who are acutely allergic to egg. Recent studies have shown that the measles vaccine can be safely given to children with egg allergy but caution is still advised. Immunisation should be carried out under supervised conditions.

Feature	Autoimmune CAH	Hepatitis B & C associated CAH
% all cases of CAH in the UK	50–80%	20–50%
Sex	85% female	Male preponderance
Associated extrahepatic autoimmune disease	Common	Rare
Smooth muscle antibodies	Positive in 70%	Low or absent
ANA	Positive in 80%	Negative
Anti-DNA antibodies	May be positive	Negative
Antimitochondrial antibodies	Positive in 25%	Negative
Antibodies to liver and kidney microsomes	May be positive	Yes (especially children)
Serum immunoglobulins	IgG ++	Normal/IgG+
HLA type	HLA B8,-DR3	–
Response to corticosteroids	Good	Not indicated
Response to IFNα	Not indicated	Good
Risk of hepatoma	Low	Significant

Adapted from Chapel and Haeney, Essentials of Clinical Immunology, 3rd edn, Blackwells, 12.11

Appendix 5 Major differences between the two main types of chronic active hepatitis (CAH).

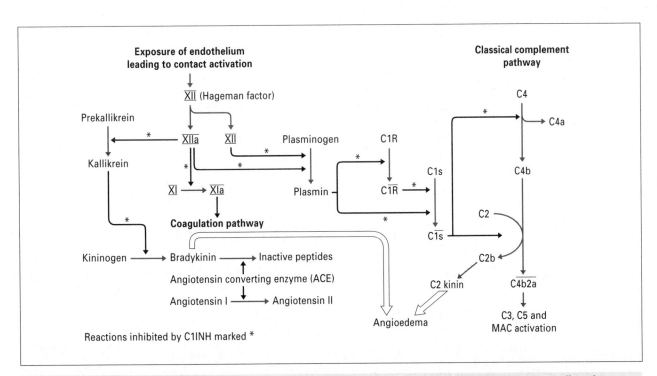

Appendix 6 Angioedema can be a life-threatening result of C1INH deficiency. However this clinical result can also be an effect of angiotensin-converting enzyme inhibitors (ACEIs), for example, captopril and enalapril. The exact mechanism of ACEI mediated angioedema is not clear but they do block the conversion of angiotensin I to angiotensin II and also inhibit the breakdown of bradykinin. Care must be taken with patients taking ACEIs who complain of angioedema.

Pre-formed mediators		De novo synthesised mediators					
Mediator	Functions	Mediator	Broncho-constriction	Vasomotor tone	Platelet accumulation	Vascular permeability	Neutrophil chemotaxis
Histamine	• Contraction of smooth muscle in airway & gut • Vasodilatation • Microvascular leakage	PGD$_2$	++	↓	−	↑	+
		PGF$_2$	++	↓	−	↓	−
Tryptase	• Cleaves fibrinogen • Promotes C3 C3a • Activates fibroblasts	TXA$_2$	++	↑	+	↓	−
		LTB$_4$	−	↓	−	↑	+
Eosinophil chemotactic factor	• Eosinophil chemotaxis and activation	LTC$_4$	++	↑	−	↑	−
Neutrophil chemotactic factor	• Neutrophil chemotaxis and activation	LTD$_4$	++	↓	−	↑	−
Heparin	• Anticoagulant • Fibrinolytic • Anticomplement	LTE$_4$	+	↓	−	↑	−
		PAF	+	↑	+	↑	+

Interleukins
  IL-3
  IL-4
  IL-5
  IL-6
  TNFα
	• Promotion of the IgE response						

PG = prostaglandin; TX = thromboxane; LT = leukotriene; PAF = platelet activating factor

Appendix 7 Role of mediators in allergic disease. Some cytokines enhance and promote the IgE and allergic response; interleukin (IL)-3, IL-4, IL-5, IL-6, IL-13, and tumour necrosis factor (TNF)α.

CD	Identify/function	Main cell types expressing
CD1	Unknown	Cortical thymocytes
CD2	LFA-3 receptor	Mature T cells
CD3	T-cell receptor	Mature T cells
CD4	MHC class II receptor	T-cell subset
CD5	CD72 receptor	T cells; B-cell subset
CD8	MHC class I receptor	T-cell subset
CD11α	LFA-1 (α chain)	All leucocytes
CD11β	CR3 = Mac1 (α chain)	Monocyte/macrophage neutrophil
CD14	LPS receptor	Monocyte/macrophage
CD15	Binds ELAM-1	Macrophage; granulocyte
CD16	Fcγ receptor (type III)	Phagocytes; platelets; LGLs
CD18	LFA-1 and CR3 (β chain)	All leucocytes
CD21	CR2 complement receptor	B-cell subset
CD23	Fcε receptor (low affinity)	B-cell subset
CD25	IL-2 receptor	Activated T or B cell
CD29	VLA-integrins (β chain)	All leucocytes
CD32	Fcγ receptor (type II)	B cell; mononuclear phagocytes
CD35	CR1 complement receptor	B cell; mononuclear phagocytes
CD45	Leucocyte common antigen	All leucocytes
CD45R	Restricted LCA	T-cell subsets; other leucocytes
CD46	MCP	All leucocytes
CD49α–φ	VLA-integrins (α chains)	Variable
CD54	ICAM-1	Activated leucocytes
CD55	DAF	All leucocytes
CD56	NCAM	LGLs; activated lymphocytes
CD58	LFA-3 (CD2 receptor)	All leucocytes
CD64	Fcγ receptor (type I)	Mononuclear phagocytes
CD71	Transferrin receptor	Activated lymphocyte; macrophage
CD72	CD5 receptor	B cells

CR: complement receptor; DAF: decay accelerating factor; ELAM-1: endothelial leucocyte adhesion molecule; ICAM: intercellular adhesion molecule; LFA: lymphocyte functional antigen; LPS: lipopolysaccharide; MCP: membrane cofactor protein; NCAM: neural cell adhesion molecule; VLA: very late antigen.

Appendix 8 Principal CD markers.

Cytokines	Sources	Targets	Main effects
IL-1α	Macrophages Lymphocytes Epithelium	Lymphocytes Macrophages Fibroblasts	Pro-inflammatory Cytokine production; endothelial activation Cytokine receptor induction
IL-1β	Astrocytes	Endothelium	Phagocyte activation
IL-2	T cells	T cells B cells	Required for division
IL-4	T cells	B cells	Required for division and differentiation
IL-5	T cells	B cells	Required for division and differentiation
IL-6	Macrophages Fibroblasts T cells Endothelium	T cells B cells Hepatocytes Other cells	Promote differentiation Acute phase proteins Pro-inflammatory
IL-10	T-cell subset	T-cell subset	Blocks cytokine production
IFNγ	T cells	Macrophages Other cells Endothelium	Activation MHC induction Activation
TNFα	Macrophages Lymphocytes	Lymphocytes Monocytes Natural killer cells	Activation Enhances cytotoxicity
TNFβ	T cells	Endothelium	Activation; pro-inflammatory
TGFβ	T cells B cells	T cells B cells	Inhibits activation

Appendix 9 Principal cytokines. There are now more than 17 interleukins (ILs) described.

Group	Findings
I	Acute infection associated with seroconversion
II	Asymptomatic infection (includes HIV related thrombocytopaenia)
III	Persistent generalised lymphadenopathy
IV	SYMPTOMATIC DISEASE
IV A	Constitutional disease. Any two of: • Weight loss >10% baseline • Fever >15 days in 1 month • Diarrhoea >1 month
IV B	Neurological disease caused by HIV: Encephalopathy Myelopathy Peripheral neuropathy
IV C1	Major opportunistic infections: Oesophageal candidiasis *Pneumocystis carinii* pneumonia (PCP) Cerebral toxoplasmosis Cryptococcal meningitis Cytomegalovirus (CMV) retinitis *Mycobacterium avium intracellulare* (MAI) Cryptosporidium associated diarrhoea *Mycobacterium tuberculosis* Recurrent pneumonia
IV C2	Minor opportunistic infections: Oral hairy leukoplakia (Epstein-Barr virus) Dermal herpes zoster Oral *Candida*
IV D	Cancer secondary to HIV: Kaposi's sarcoma Primary cerebral lymphoma Non–Hodgkins B-cell lymphoma Invasive cervical carcinoma
IV E	Conditions attributed to HIV infection (but not classified above): Skin conditions, e.g. seborrhoeic dermatitis Constitutional symptoms not meeting IV A Other infections, e.g. mouth ulcers
Disease progression	Seroconversion Asymptomatic PGL AIDS-related complex = IV C2 AIDS = IV A, IV C1, IV D & encephalopathy

Appendix 10 CDC classification of HIV disease.

CD4 lymphocyte count/mm³	Complications
250–500	Oral *Candida* Tuberculosis
150–200	Kaposi's sarcoma Lymphoma Cryptosporidiosis
75–125	*Pneumocystis carinii* pneumonia Toxoplasmosis Cryptococcal meningitis *Mycobacterium avium* complex Recurrent herpes simplex ulceration Oesophageal *Candida*
<50	Cytomegalovirus retinitis

Appendix 11 HIV: CD4 lymphocyte counts and clinical complications.

A

AAE	Acquired angioedema
ABPA	Allergic bronchopulmonary aspergillosis
ACE	Angiotensin converting enzyme
Ach	Acetylcholine
AchR	Acetylcholine receptor
ACTH	Adrenocorticotrophic hormone
AIDS	Acquired immunodeficiency syndrome
AIHA	Autoimmune haemolytic anaemia
ALL	Acute lymphoblastic leukaemia
AML	Acute myeloid leukaemia
ANCA	Antineutrophil cytoplasmic antibody
AP	Anterior–posterior
APC	Antigen presenting cell
APTT	Activated partial thromboplastin time
ARDS	Adult respiratory distress syndrome
AS	Ankylosing spondylitis
ASGP-R	Asialoglycoprotein receptor

B

BAL	Bronchoalveolar lavage
btk	Bruton's tyrosine kinase

C

C1INH	C1 inhibitor
CAH	Chronic active hepatitis
CGD	Chronic granulomatous disease
CHAD	Cold haemagglutinin disease
CMV	Cytomegalovirus
CREST	Calcinosis, Raynaud's, esophageal, sclerodactyly, telangiectasia
CRP	C reactive protein
CSF	Cerebrospinal fluid

D

DAT	Direct antiglobulin test
DIC	Disseminated intravascular coagulation

E

EAA	Extrinsic allergic alveolitis
EAM	External auditory meatus
EBV	Epstein–Barr virus
ELISA	Enzyme-linked immunosorbent assay
ESR	Erythrocyte sedimentation rate

F

FEV1	Forced expiratory volume in 1 second
FS	Felty's syndrome
FVC	Forced vital capacity

G

GAD	Glutamic acid decarboxylase
GBM	Glomerular basement membrane
GM-CSF	Granulocyte–macrophage colony stimulating factors

H

HAE	Hereditary angioedema
HDN	Haemolytic disease of the newborn
HLA	Human leucocyte antigen
HSV	Herpes simplex virus

I

IDDM	Insulin dependent diabetes mellitus
IL	Interleukin

L

LKM	Liver/kidney/microsomal antibody
LSP	Liver-specific membrane lipoprotein

M

MAC	Membrane attack complex
MBP	Major basic protein
MCHC	Mean cell haemoglobin concentration
MCV	Mean cell volume
MCH	Mean cell haemoglobin
MHC	Major histocompatibility complex

N

NBT	Nitroblue tetrazolium test
NSAID	Non-steroidal anti-inflammatory drug

O

osp A	Outer surface protein A

P

PAF	Platelet activating factor
PALS	Periarteriolar lymphoid sheath
PCH	Paroxysmal cold haemoglobinuria
PCP	*Pneumocystis carinii* pneumonia
PCR	Polymerase chain reaction
PG	Prostaglandin
PHA	Phytohaemagglutinin
PTH	Parathyroid hormone

R

RAST	Radioallergosorbent test

S

SMA	Smooth muscle antibody

T

TIBC	Total iron binding capacity
TNF	Tumour necrosis factor

V

VSV	Vesicular stomatitis virus

Index

Letters in bold refer to figures